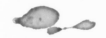

# PICKLES & ICE CREAM

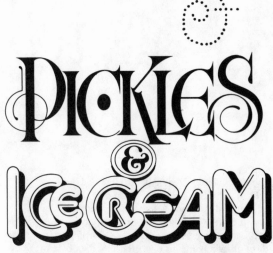

# PICKLES & ICE CREAM

## The Complete Guide to Nutrition During Pregnancy

Mary Abbott Hess, R.D., M.S.
Anne Elise Hunt

Foreword by Roy M. Pitkin, M.D.
Illustrations by Keith J. Taylor

McGRAW-HILL BOOK COMPANY

New York   St. Louis   San Francisco
Hamburg   Mexico   Toronto

Copyright © 1982 by Mary Abbott Hess and Anne
Elise Hunt. All rights reserved. Printed in the
United States of America. Except as permitted under
the United States Copyright Act of 1976, no part of
this publication may be reproduced or distributed in
any form or by any means or stored in a data base or
retrieval system, without the prior written permission
of the publisher.

1 2 3 4 5 6 7 8 9 B P B P 8 7 6 5 4 3 2

ISBN 0-07-028419-9

LIBRARY OF CONGRESS CATALOGING IN PUBLICATION DATA

Hess, Mary Abbott.
Pickles and ice cream.
Bibliography: p.
1. Pregnancy—Nutritional aspects.
I. Hunt, Anne Elise. II. Title.
RG559.H47        618.2'4        81-20824
ISBN 0-07-028419-9          AACR2

Book design by Roberta Rezk

This book is not intended to replace the services of a
physician. Any application of the recommendations
set forth in the following pages is at the reader's
discretion and sole risk.

## Consulting Authorities

**Carole Chambers, Ph.D.**                     Chapters 3, 11

*Associate Professor*
Mundelein College, Chicago

**Harriet Danzyger, R.D.**                     Chapters 7, 10

*Clinical Dietitian*
Northwestern Memorial Hospital
Prentice Women's Hospital and Maternity Center, Chicago

**Deborah V. Edidin, M.D.**                    Chapters 3, 4, 5

*Assistant Professor of Pediatrics*
Pritzker School of Medicine
University of Chicago

*Attending Physician*
*Department of Pediatrics*
Division of Endocrinology
Kunstadter Childrens Center
Michael Reese Hospital and Medical Center, Chicago

**Marilyn C. Frederiksen, M.D.**            **Chapters 6, 9**

*Specialist in Maternal-Fetal Medicine*
Northwestern Memorial Hospital
Prentice Women's Hospital and Maternity Center, Chicago

**Mary Hughes, Ph.D.**            **Chapter 8**

*Vice President for Public Health Education*
March of Dimes Birth Defects Foundation

**Howard N. Jacobson, M.D.**            **Chapters 1-11**

*Director, Institute of Nutrition*
University of North Carolina

**Edward Ogata, M.D.**            **Chapter 4**

*Attending Neonatologist*
Northwestern Memorial Hospital
Prentice Women's Hospital and Maternity Center, Chicago

*Assistant Professor of Obstetrics and Gynecology*
Northwestern University Medical School, Chicago

**Roy M. Pitkin, M.D.**            **Chapters 1–11**

*Chairman, Department of Obstetrics
and Gynecology*
University of Iowa

**Laura Zell Vitt**            **Chapter 11**

*Coordinator, Health Learning Center*
Northwestern Memorial Hospital, Chicago

# Contents

# Foreword

Nutrition during pregnancy is a topic of great contemporary interest, based on the assumption that maternal nutritional status represents a foundation upon which rests the health and well-being of future generations. With the recent trend toward fewer children per family has come increasing concern with the quality of life of each child and pregnancy nutrition is widely and logically regarded as an important determinant of that quality.

One of several encouraging characteristics of the current generation of women of childbearing age is a deep and consuming interest in understanding factors which influence the health of themselves and their children. Today's woman wants to know as much as possible about these matters and she expects, indeed even demands, that her information be accurate and understandable. Mary Abbott Hess and Anne Elise Hunt have met this need admirably in a treatment of the subject that is as accurate as it is thorough, as comprehensive as it is systematic, as practical as it is informative. Its style is an eminently readable one and the illustrations by Keith J. Taylor are a delight.

Hess and Hunt, while documenting the importance of pregnancy nutrition with the most recent of scientific research and thought, have not lost sight of the fact that eating is also one of the more enjoyable of social customs. They have been careful to emphasize that food is not medicine, diet not a panacea, and nutrition not a talisman.

As a physician, I will find this book of great value in the care of my patients. Women will find it helpful in their quest to make informed choices about their health and that of their families. But perhaps the greatest beneficiaries will be those "generations yet unborn."

ROY M. PITKIN, M.D.

# PICKLES & ICE CREAM

# Introduction

What is the *most important* to you?
1. To have a daughter.
2. To have a son.
3. To have a healthy baby.

Most women choose 3, To have a healthy baby. In this book, we are going to show you the best way to prepare for that healthy baby.

Fortunately, most babies are born healthy, but it doesn't just happen. Many factors determine the outcome of pregnancy. Some of these factors—for example, your age—you cannot control; but others, such as regular medical care and the food you eat, depend on decisions that you make.

You may be one of many women today who have a serious interest in nutrition. You are concerned about whether your diet is adequate now that you are pregnant. On the other hand,

1

you may not have given much thought to nutrition before you became pregnant. Now you want to be sure to eat what is best for your developing child. Every one has heard "pickles and ice cream" stories about pregnancy. While pickles and ice cream, even together, won't hurt you, they are not the best foundation for a prenatal diet.

There are many books about pregnancy, but few deal specifically with nutrition in a comprehensive, responsible way. This book will help you make better choices about what to eat and drink. We have included the most recent findings about substances that can interfere with the development of your baby. We will tell you what is good for you and baby, too!

Mary is a registered dietitian and former nutrition professor. Many women have come to her seeking nutritional guidance when they became pregnant. "They want information about nutrition in clear, non-technical language. They want to understand how their baby is developing. They want to make informal decisions about food based on facts and their own values. They often want to know about my experiences when I was pregnant. They want to know about risks and dangers."

The book became a reality when Mary Abbott Hess and Anne Hunt became partners. Anne has a dual career of mother/food journalist. Her skills provided an added dimension: "What you eat should bring you comfort and a sense of pleasure, as well as health. If we are going to write about nutrition during pregnancy, we shouldn't make it sound like a nine-month ordeal at the dinner table!"

Before writing the book, we reviewed hundreds of articles in current journals of obstetrics, nursing, and nutrition, and read background material in many textbooks. We drew from newspapers and magazines, attended lectures and presentations, conducted telephone interviews with professionals, and listened to tapes on the subject.

We worked together until Anne, who does not have a technical background, could understand it, and Mary, who knows all the "right" words, said it was accurate. We then sent each chapter to doctors, dietitians, or professional organizations for expert review.

The book is more than technically correct; it is an accurate account of how women experience pregnancy. We have shared our own experiences and those of our families and friends. It took us nine months to write the book. We hope that our "labor" helps you to have a better pregnancy and a healthy baby.

# 1.
# What Good Nutrition Will and Will Not Do

Anyone who has raised plants from seed knows that there is more to it than the directions on the package lead you to believe: "Sow the seed outdoors in the spring after the soil is warm and all danger of frost is past. Sow in a sunny location. Cover with ¼" fine soil. Height, 1½ feet."

If seeds are to grow to their maximum height and bloom, conditioning of the soil, providing space between young plants, regular watering and occasional fertilizing, and careful attention to disease prevention are necessary. Prize-winning plants rarely "just happen."

When we learned about making babies back in fifth-grade sex education class (discreetly called "family life" or "biology" in our school system), we were told that the father planted the seed in the mother and it grew into a baby. Sounds even simpler than the directions on the back of the garden seed packet! But if you are planning to have a baby, or are already pregnant, it's time for a few lessons in "baby horticulture."

You would think that by now, this baby-growing business would be an exact science, especially when you consider the scientific and technological methods used for successfully breeding many animals. But since we cannot conduct controlled experiments with human life, many judgments about

5

human babies must be based on observations. Unlike those of experimental animals, where environment and foods can be strictly controlled, every human pregnancy is unique and there are thousands of variables.

Fortunately, most babies are born healthy. But some babies are born less than perfect. Discouraging statistics in this country in recent years have led researchers to take a hard look at our birthing practices. The consensus is that maternal nutrition is a critical factor that too frequently has been ignored. Sometimes this has led to unfortunate consequences for both mother and baby.

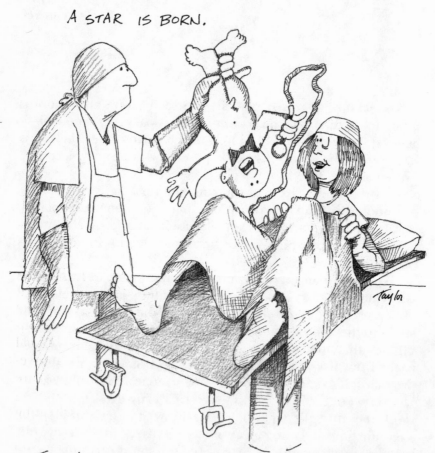

A STAR IS BORN.

FIRST I'D LIKE TO THANK MY MOM. IT'S BEEN GREAT THE LAST NINE MONTHS. THE FOOD, THE ATMOSPHERE . . . MOM, YOU'RE REALLY TERRIFIC!

There are a lot of "pickles and ice cream" ideas about maternal nutrition, but the reality is that few mothers-to-be understand the way in which their food choices and lifestyles affect their babies.

Some believe that cravings are signals from the womb demanding specific nutrients needed by the baby. Others think that the baby will get what it needs, regardless of the mother's diet. Until recently, there has been wide acceptance of the concept that the fetus is a parasite, whose needs take priority over the needs of the "host" (or in this case, "hostess").

In fact, when a mother-to-be is not getting an adequate diet, she and her baby will compete for available nutrients. When they finish dividing up their "meal," they both turn to whatever reserves there are in the mother's body to compensate for what they are missing. In the long run, neither of them gets sufficient nourishment and both are "short-changed."

Yet Mother Nature does step in to help! There are changes that take place during pregnancy that help to protect the baby with minimum risks to the mother. During pregnancy, many nutrients are absorbed more efficiently so that maternal stores are increased and the baby's needs can be met.

But if the quality and quantity of the mother's diet are adequate, both before conception and during pregnancy, most women will experience fewer complications during pregnancy and labor and deliver larger, healthier babies. The mother's recovery is faster and breastfeeding is more likely to be successful.

To be useful, any advice related to health should be tailored to the individual. To help you make informed decisions about your pregnancy, you must first determine your nutritional status. Throughout this book, there will be short questionnaires and quizzes to help you look at your own nutritional habits, spot strengths, and learn the areas that need improvement. The answers, when there are right and wrong ones, are found on page 233.

If you enter pregnancy with well-established good eating habits, you will find that you will have to make very few changes; if your eating patterns are now irregular or poor, you can modify your habits to improve your own health and that of your baby.

# PRELIMINARY INVENTORY

*Vital Statistics:*

Age:
Height:
Due date:
Weight before pregnancy:
Have you ever had any problems with your weight? If so, describe:



*Health History:*

Do you have any health problems? If so, describe:


Are you under care for these problems?


Have you ever had a nutrition-related illness, such as anemia?


*Nutrition Habits:*

Do you eat at regular mealtimes?
How many meals do you eat each day?
Do you eat breakfast?
Do you eat differently on weekends than on weekdays?
Describe:


Do you frequently eat away from home (cafeteria, brown-bag lunch, restaurants)? Describe:


Are you on any special diet (diabetic, vegetarian, weight-loss, hypoglycemic, etc.)? Describe:

Do you take any vitamin supplements? If yes, what?

Do you think you have good eating habits?

*Previous Pregnancies:*

Have you been pregnant before?
How many times have you been pregnant prior to this
pregnancy?
How long ago was your last pregnancy?
How much weight did you gain during your last completed
pregnancy?
Did you experience any complications during your previous
pregnancy?
If so, describe:

*Physical Activity:*

Do you consider yourself physically active?

What types of exercise do you prefer?

How many times a week do you have sustained physical
exercise lasting at least 20 minutes?

## Assessing Your Nutritional Status

### Age

Biologically speaking, a "mature woman" is eighteen to thirty-five years old—prime time for meeting the biological challenges of pregnancy. Twenty to twenty-nine are the "bonus baby" years, statistically the *most* successful time for pregnancy.

Not that this has discouraged women at either end of the spectrum. One out of every four mothers in the United States, bearing her first child is under twenty years old. And, according to the National Center for Health Statistics, in recent years there has been a 22 percent increase in births to women thirty-five to thirty-nine years old. It isn't unusual these days for women in their early forties to bear children.

How can nutritional management help minimize problems?

■ *The Younger Woman* Nearly a third of a girl's total growth, half her weight, and 10 to 15 percent of her height are gained during adolescence. This accelerated growth demands a strong and steady supply of nutrients. Pregnancy makes enormous additional demands that are hard to meet. Babies born to women whose own bodies are still growing run the risk of being nutritionally shortchanged.

A young woman's lifestyle is frequently not designed for meeting the demands of pregnancy. Meals may be infrequent and/or irregular, heavy on fries and soft drinks, easy on fresh fruits and vegetables and milk. There may be experimentation with alcohol, cigarettes, and drugs. There is a high incidence of infection, especially among those whose diets are marginal. This is a difficult environment for growing babies!

If you are under eighteen and pregnant, you will want to make a special effort to eat an adequate diet. What you do now will not only help avoid complications during your pregnancy; it can also have a lifetime effect on both you and your baby. Babies born to teenage mothers tend to have lower birth weights than the babies of older women. Low-birth-weight babies have a decreased chance for survival and a greater chance of mental and physical handicaps. Some of these babies never catch up as they grow up. Women in this age group *can* produce excellent normal-birth-weight babies, but it does take extra effort.

Agnes Higgins, director of the Montreal Diet Dispensary, a clinic for low-income pregnant women in Montreal, Canada, has had great success working with young mothers. Eighty percent of the women who enter her clinic are found to have poor nutritional status. This condition is not exclusive to the poor; many women, regardless of social or economic situation, are poorly nourished. The Montreal Diet Dispensary has demonstrated that simply adding to the diet milk, eggs, and oranges, and a vitamin and mineral supplement—with no other changes—can have a dramatic effect on the outcome of pregnancy.[88]

Mrs. Higgins points out that the pregnant woman is really "eating for two." If you want your baby to grow, you must feed it the proper food every day—before it is born, as well as after.

The techniques used by the Montreal Diet Dispensary have been so successful that the March of Dimes Birth Defects Foundation has created the Agnes Higgins Award, which is given to those who make outstanding contributions in the field of maternal and fetal nutrition.

■ *The Older Woman* Statistics indicate that women over thirty have a greater number of complications in pregnancy than do younger mothers. Current studies indicate that supporting a growing fetus becomes more difficult as a woman gets older and her body is less able to adjust to change, but there are few studies that have probed the underlying causes. As more women elect to have babies later in life, research will ascertain the specific changes occurring after the peak childbearing years that affect pregnancy. Individual experiences do vary greatly; it was recently reported that a Russian woman had given birth in her sixties.

It isn't just teenagers whose lifestyle during pregnancy may put them at risk. The "over-thirty moms" have their own set of lifestyle problems. If you are in this age group, you surely have well-established eating and lifestyle patterns that you may find yourself very reluctant to change. Not that you mind fruits and vegetables, but how do you feel about trading your evening glass of wine with dinner for milk? Or cutting back on coffee? And, after all these years of watching your figure, you may be reluctant to go with the current recommendations for weight gain.

Busy women may have eating patterns that are as unsound as those of many sixteen-year-olds. How many times have you started the day with only a cup of coffee, then had a high calorie doughnut mid-morning to stave off hunger pangs?

Several of Mary's close friends are women who have decided, after the age of thirty-five, to have their first child. Some are professional women who "reconsider" their decision not to have children as they approach their fortieth birthday; others delay making the decision—and then it is a now-or-never situation! Most of these women who have become pregnant had amniocentesis to determine that their fetuses did not have the birth defects that are more prevalent among babies of older moms. There has been the usual range of minor pregnancy problems. Several women have said that they tire very easily, and rest periods are essential. But this isn't unique to the older mother. Most of these women are quite concerned with their diet and are willing to do whatever is necessary to have the best chance of having a healthy baby. This motivation more than compensates for the poorly understood differences in physiologic functioning of the older mom.

Jonathan, Judy Wise's son, was born the week of her fortieth birthday. "There's so much about pregnancy that is outside your control that it felt very important to me to take care with those few things I could have impact on. So I was very careful about what I put in my body and I felt that I was doing what I could to contribute to my own and my baby's health and well-being."

## Previous Nutritional Status

■ *You Are What Your Mother Ate* There are women who are short (5'1" or less) or thin because they come from families where this is a genetic trait. There are also women whose small stature may have been influenced by their nutritional histories. Even before birth, their bodies were being shaped; if their mothers were poorly nourished during pregnancy, their daughters may be smaller than genetics would predict. Many babies are born with lifelong potential for frail bones and weak teeth because their mothers did not choose calcium-rich foods, or drink fluoridated water. Without modifications that improve your diet, you may be perpetuating this cycle.

■ *You Are What You Ate* Before you put all the blame on what your mother ate when she was carrying you, take a good look at your own eating habits. It may be that in spite of persistent urgings to eat your breakfast, or take a sandwich to eat at lunch instead of a candy bar, you went right ahead and did as you pleased as you were growing up.

If you have always been concerned about your figure (and you certainly aren't alone!), you may have tried a number of fad diets over the years, avoided milk because you thought it fattening, or skipped meals when you "felt fat." If you began these practices during adolescence, you may not now have good reserves of those nutrients that can be stored for periods of physiologic stress—such as pregnancy.

Statistically, women whose physique suggests nutritional negligence prior to pregnancy have a greater number of miscarriages, stillbirths, and delivery complications. Their babies are shorter and weigh less than babies born to mothers with adequate diets. The implication is that a good diet prior to pregnancy is one of the factors in determining the outcome of pregnancy. But good nutrition during pregnancy, as the Montreal Diet Dispensary program and other studies have shown, can reduce complications during pregnancy and increase the size and potential of the baby.

## Weight: Over and Under

■ *The underweight woman should make every effort before and during her pregnancy to achieve her ideal body weight and then gain extra pounds for pregnancy.* This means that she should gain weight far in excess of what would normally be gained during pregnancy. For some women, this is very difficult to do.

If you are overweight or obese, you probably can't even imagine the problems just described. Your problem is how to deal with additional weight gain in pregnancy. Ideally, you should have lost any excess weight before you became pregnant. A few pounds doesn't matter, but extreme obesity contributes to medical problems and a more difficult delivery.

■ *More-than-adequate weight doesn't necessarily mean adequate nutrition.* In fact, many overweight women are suffering from *under*nutrition. Babies need more than fat to grow. Body fat can be the result of excessive calories from fats, sugars, or alcohol—all poor sources of necessary vitamins and minerals. Body fat cannot break down to yield protein and the other nutrients that you need during pregnancy. So you will need to make food choices that will provide the essential nutrients that you and your baby need. If you are obese, you will want to work closely with your doctor throughout your pregnancy. You can deal with your weight problem after your delivery. *Pregnancy is not the time for a restricted diet.*

> *The American College of Obstetricians and Gynecologists warns that any attempt to restrict your diet during pregnancy, even if you are overweight, can jeopardize your baby.*

■ *What a Difference a Sperm Makes!* The inventory you completed asked about your eating habits. Irregular eating—such as skipping meals, or having a quick snack at your desk or at the kitchen table instead of eating lunch—may be your lifestyle, but it is not the lifestuff of which babies are made. Knowing how much it affects the kind of baby you produce will help you to reevaluate and make changes now.

Your baby needs a constant supply of high-quality nutrients to develop into a healthy human being. Recent studies show that children of mothers who fasted or skipped meals during pregnancy did less well on IQ tests at age four than children of mothers with regular eating habits.[61]

If you have been on a special diet, now is the time to examine it to see if it meets your needs during pregnancy. If you are a vegetarian, some adjustments will be necessary. If you have an existing medical problem, you will need additional prenatal care to meet both your medical and nutritional needs.

### Previous Pregnancies

■ *How Many? How Often? How Big?* If you have had difficulty with previous pregnancies, you may be anxious to know if there are ways that nutrition can improve the situation.

Very recent studies show that women who have a greater percentage of lean body weight, as compared to fat stores, may have trouble conceiving. The body seems to need some nutritional reserves in the form of stored fat. Those who are very active in athletics, such as marathon runners and swimmers, tend to be most commonly affected as they may have depleted nutrient reserves even if their diet is quite good.

A woman who has had three or more pregnancies within a few years has put an enormous strain on her body and her nutrient stores. It takes several months for her body to recover after pregnancy and be in optimal condition to bear another child. Even the farmer gives the land a chance to rest between crops! If you are still breastfeeding, or have recently finished breastfeeding, those nutrients that can be stored may be depleted.

The amount and pattern of your weight gain during previous pregnancies and the birth weight of your babies may be indicators of potential nutrition-related problems. If your children have been unusually heavy at birth, your doctor will be especially watchful for latent diabetes mellitus.

If you have had a history of obstetrical problems, you will want to explore every possible means to improve the outcome. Good nutrition is not a guarantee of a perfect pregnancy; but good food choices can be thought of as an insurance policy against many problems that you and baby could encounter if your food choices were more casual.

### What About Twins?

There are a number of factors involved in the development of twins that you cannot control. Twins are limited in size by the potential of the placenta and the degree to which the uterus can expand. Add to this your age, pre-pregnancy status, and genetic factors. Often twins are born prematurely. They need all the help they can get, especially if they begin life outside the womb several weeks earlier than other babies. Your doctor will monitor your pregnancy carefully and help you determine appropriate levels of nutrients. Though some of the numbers may vary, the information in this book still applies.

## The Stress Factor

Stress occurs any time there are changes or threats that require a physical or emotional response. There is physical stress during pregnancy as your growing baby makes demands on you, both physically and emotionally. Most mothers-to-be experience some stress as they think about the changes a baby will bring about in their lifestyle. Even positive stress, such as the anticipation and excitement you feel when you think about the baby coming, causes a physical and emotional reaction. This is normal, and can be handled by your body.

If something happens during your pregnancy that brings about unusual stress, such as loss of a job, moving, or a death in the family, both you and your baby will be affected. Stress acts on your body in strange ways. One of the most obvious reactions to stress is a change in appetite. Some people lose their appetite while others eat great quantities of "comfort foods," which may interfere with good nutritional patterns. Stress alters levels of hormones that affect the absorption and utilization of nutrients.[134] The well-nourished person is better able to cope with the nutritional demands imposed by stress.

You can help yourself by finding understanding friends, relatives, or professionals with whom you can talk. Find activities that will help you cope with frustration and tension. Exercises taught in prenatal classes may help you to relax; many women enjoy yoga, meditation, aerobic dancing, or other forms of exercise.

Through it all, you need to remember to take good care of your baby. This is not a time to seek relief from stress or tension by taking tranquilizers or alcohol, which can harm your baby. Even though you may not feel like eating at all, your baby is depending on you for daily nourishment.

## Eight Hours of Sleep and Long Walks

Physical conditioning is as important to good health during pregnancy as it is when you are not pregnant. A regular program of exercise will increase your sense of well-being—both physical and emotional.

If you are in good health, and have been physically active

prior to pregnancy, you can probably continue your regular exercise during pregnancy, except where balance is involved or when there is a chance that you may fall.

Our friend Jacqueline Marcus jogged several miles every day, including the morning she went into labor. She said that jogging felt better than walking, because it relieved the pressure and the baby seemed to be floating. We are not necessarily recommending this to you. Jackie was in great physical shape before pregnancy and is participating in a research study on the effects of exercise in pregnancy.

The last months of pregnancy put a great strain on your circulatory system. If you do strenuous physical exercise or work, your muscles will compete with the placenta for blood, straining your heart; if you have not had previous physical conditioning, this risks premature delivery. Your doctor will help you to determine an appropriate program of physical activity for your pregnancy.

Physical activity can improve your appetite, reduce stress, and help you sleep better during pregnancy. "R and R," as they say in the military (rest and recreation), is especially important. It is wise to sleep at least eight hours a night and have several rest periods, however brief, during the day. Mary loved her late-afternoon naps after work and before dinner and evening activities. Take a little time with your feet up to regenerate. Exercise, rest, relaxation, and nutrition all play important roles during pregnancy.

The scope of this book does not allow us to discuss specific exercise programs during pregnancy. There are a number of excellent books available, and a variety of exercise classes are offered in most communities. Healthy pregnant women have come out of the closet and are dancing, stretching, running, skiing, and walking to the delivery room.

## Identifying the Risk Factors

Every mother needs prenatal care beginning early in her pregnancy. Some obstetricians and family physicians place more emphasis on nutrition than do others. In any case, your food choices will ultimately be the result of *your* actions.

> *This book is designed to give you the information that you need to make informed choices, but it will not substitute for good medical care.*

Pregnancy is a normal condition. Under most circumstances, babies will grow and flourish if given proper nurturing. There are situations that require nutritional modifications. You can use this book as a guide if you

* need to know how to eat better to improve the outcome of your pregnancy
* are concerned about the quality of your diet
* have irregular eating patterns
* are unsure about eating "convenience foods" when you are pregnant
* are a vegetarian
* are underweight
* are overweight, but not obese
* smoke
* drink alcoholic beverages
* suffer from stress (provided it is not severe).

Other situations, including almost all medical complications, require the guidance of a professional with training in therapeutic nutrition in addition to your regular medical care. If you need nutrition counseling, your doctor can refer you to a registered dietitian, a nutrition clinic at the hospital, a public health nutritionist, or a nutritionist with a community health program. Many doctors prefer to provide the nutrition counseling you need themselves.

Feel free to ask questions and keep a question list between appointments with your doctor or nutrition counselor. We hope that this book will help you to know what questions to ask and to better understand the answers.

# 2.
# Having a Baby:
# A Weighty Subject

How much do you know about weight control in pregnancy?
Answer these questions and then read this chapter. The correct
answers are on page 233.

**True or False**

_____ 1. Overweight women are almost always well
nourished.

_____ 2. It is dangerous to the baby if the mother fasts
or regularly skips meals during pregnancy.

_____ 3. In the first three months of pregnancy, a
typical weight gain is about 4 pounds.

_____ 4. Babies born weighing from 5 to 7 pounds are
generally healthier than babies weighing
from 7 to 9 pounds.

_____ 5. If a pregnant woman gains over 3 pounds in
one week, she should call her doctor.

_____ 6. A healthy weight gain during pregnancy for a

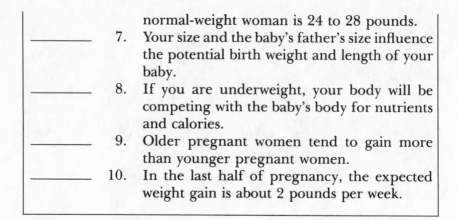

normal-weight woman is 24 to 28 pounds.

_____ 7. Your size and the baby's father's size influence the potential birth weight and length of your baby.

_____ 8. If you are underweight, your body will be competing with the baby's body for nutrients and calories.

_____ 9. Older pregnant women tend to gain more than younger pregnant women.

_____ 10. In the last half of pregnancy, the expected weight gain is about 2 pounds per week.

After you've announced to your friends and family that you are expecting a baby, you will begin to receive all sorts of advice and counsel about pregnancy—especially about how much weight you should gain.

If you are one of those women who has worked very hard to maintain a slim figure, you are probably concerned about getting into your clothes after the baby is born. On the other hand, if you are a little overweight you may be thinking that—since you will be watching your diet anyway during your pregnancy—this would be a good opportunity to lose a few pounds so you will be "back to normal" after the baby. Overweight women may be reluctant to gain any additional weight. If you're working you are, no doubt, increasingly aware of the unpregnant shapes in your office, and you may not want to appear "dowdy" by comparison.

As a responsible mother-to-be, you want to know how much weight you should gain to produce a healthy baby, and at the same time, you are concerned about managing this weight so your baby will have a happy and healthy mother.

Weight gain is one of the most discussed aspects of pregnancy; it is also a topic of considerable disagreement. The reason is that, like fashion, advice about weight gain during pregnancy has changed over the years to reflect the times, and not everyone you talk to is aware of the current research.

During the eighteenth century, women often suffered from a variety of nutritional deficiencies. Poorly formed bones, especially when pressed into corsets, caused women of the time to have very small pelvises. When weight gain was limited, their babies were born smaller and were easier to deliver. At that time the emphasis was on the mother, and the health and potential of the baby were seldom even considered. Virtually nothing was known about nutrition, much less about its relation to anyone's health!

In the early part of this century, large families were common. A woman indulged herself during pregnancy. If she gained a few pounds in the process, it was only a sign of her commitment to producing a family. "She's fat because, after all, she's had six children" was not an unusual or unkind evaluation.

During World War I, diets were limited by necessity. Doctors came to the conclusion that, by restricting weight gain, many complications of pregnancy could be avoided. This theory persisted for the next forty years. "Tall and thin" became the ideal of many women, and the idea of limited weight gain during pregnancy was what women wanted to hear. Weight control was stressed and women were advised not to gain "too much" weight—typically, no more than 16 to 18 pounds. In the late 1960s a weight gain of no more than 20 pounds was still advocated by many doctors and university centers.

Anne remembers, "There was never any mention of what I should eat; it was as if the only thing that mattered was not to gain more than the doctor decreed. He told me that if I couldn't exercise enough self-control to manage my weight during pregnancy, then I would not be a good mother (just what a tentative first-time mother-to-be needs to hear). On the day of my appointment, I would not eat breakfast. How I dreaded the moment when I had to get on the scale! After the exam, I would rush to the Palmer House Coffee Shop and order a huge breakfast. I was very proud that I gained only 18 pounds."

Deborah Edidin, M.D., now a pediatric endocrinologist at Michael Reese Hospital, in Chicago, remembers debating (with herself) whether or not to cancel her appointment with her obstetrician when she gained more than she was supposed to.

Until recently it was thought that the development of the fetus was unrelated to the weight of the mother, the amount she gained, or the rate at which she gained it. Current studies show that quite the opposite is true. The mother's pre-pregnancy weight and the total weight gained during pregnancy are, except for the number of fetal development days, the single most important factor in determining birth weight. (23) And birth weight, Mother, is a critical factor in getting your child off to a good start in life.

---

## BETTER BIGGER BABIES*

---

Full-term babies weighing 7 pounds or more, when compared to full-term babies weighing 5½ pounds or less—
* have fewer physical handicaps
* have a lower rate of infant mortality
* are less likely to be mentally retarded
* have higher IQs
* suffer fewer serious illnesses during childhood
* have fewer hearing and visual disorders
* have fewer behavioral problems
* are more mature and better able to handle environmental stress
* have a head start both physically and mentally over their smaller peers, who never catch up, no matter how well fed they are, how loved they are, or how stimulating their environment may be.

*Data on American infants show that average birth weights range from 6 pounds 10 ounces to 8 pounds 13 ounces. In this book, when we refer to a "normal 7-pound baby," we are referring to the range of weights as described above. Genetic potential, including the parents' size, will influence the baby's weight, and some "normal" babies may not fall within this range.

---

Unfortunately, there are no guarantees of a healthy, intelligent baby. Premature birth, genetic factors, maternal size, race, environment, and abnormal development within the womb can affect the development of the baby; so can the mother's use of drugs, alcohol, and tobacco. Babies with severe problems are sometimes born to mothers who seem to have done everything "right." Every prospective mother, and father, worries about this, for every parent wants a healthy child.

Some factors you can control; others you cannot. When you look at the list of statistical advantages favoring babies weighing at least 7 pounds, you will want to do everything that you *can* do to make it happen. There is not much you can do about your age or height, or your genetic history. On the other hand, you *can* seek early medical care and you *can* control what you eat. If you smoke or drink beverages containing alcohol, you will want to give some careful consideration to the potential dangers to your unborn child.

## How to Build a Better Baby

To determine a goal for weight gain during pregnancy, we will first look at your pre-pregnancy weight, which medically is called your *pregravid weight*. All pregnant women do not have the same needs; our preliminary evaluation, though individualized, does not take into consideration the special risks of women who have a history of problems with pregnancy, genetic disorders, hypertension, diabetes, and so on. Each woman must be carefully assessed in terms of her own health needs.

In 1959 the Metropolitan Life Insurance Company published a Table of Desirable Weights, which has been used as the standard for determining ideal weight. These tables are being revised in the light of current research, and new figures are expected some time in 1982. In the meantime, the chart on the following page will give you an estimate of what your pre-pregnancy weight should be (or should have been).

The chart on the following page is based on *frame sizes*. This means the size and density of your bone structure. Most women fall into the range of "medium frame." Look at your wrists and ankles; if they are particularly large or small as compared to those of other women of your height, you may fall into one of the other categories.

One way of determining frame size is to measure your wrist using a cloth tape measure. Garland Anderson, M.D. gives the following guidelines for determining frame size.

Many women in our society consider themselves *overweight*, even if they are well within the normal range. When we use the

## WRIST MEASUREMENT

| Height (Barefoot) | Small Frame | Medium Frame | Large Frame |
|---|---|---|---|
| Up to 5'3" | under 5½" | 5½ to 5¾" | over 5¾" |
| 5'3" to 5'4" | under 6" | 6 to 6¼" | over 6¼" |
| 5'4" or taller | under 6¼" | 6¼ to 6½" | over 6½" |

term "overweight" in this book, we are referring to the numbers in the weight table. The term *desirable weight*, sometimes called *ideal weight* or *optimal weight*, is based on life insurance statistics; that is, the healthiest range of weight for a given height. These terms have nothing to do with how you, as an individual, perceive your weight according to your self-image or society's idea of fashionable weight.

To determine your weight status, calculate the difference between your "desirable weight" and your pre-pregnancy

## DESIRABLE WEIGHTS
### Women Ages 25 and Over in Indoor Clothing

| Height (Barefoot) | Small Frame | Medium Frame | Large Frame |
|---|---|---|---|
| 5 feet | 95 | 102 | 112 |
| 5 feet 1 inch | 98 | 104 | 114 |
| 5 feet 2 inches | 100 | 107 | 117 |
| 5 feet 3 inches | 103 | 110 | 120 |
| 5 feet 4 inches | 106 | 113 | 123 |
| 5 feet 5 inches | 109 | 116 | 126 |
| 5 feet 6 inches | 112 | 120 | 130 |
| 5 feet 7 inches | 115 | 123 | 134 |
| 5 feet 8 inches | 119 | 128 | 138 |
| 5 feet 9 inches | 123 | 132 | 142 |
| 5 feet 10 inches | 127 | 136 | 146 |
| 5 feet 11 inches | 131 | 140 | 150 |
| 6 feet | 135 | 144 | 154 |

For women aged 18 to 24, subtract one pound per year under age 25.

Adapted from: Anderson, Garland D. "Nutrition in Pregnancy—1978."
*Southern Medical Journal*, 72 (October 1979):1308.

weight. The American College of Obstetricians and Gynecologists and The American Dietetic Association have determined that women at less than 85 percent of ideal weight for height, or more than 120 percent of ideal weight for height, are at increased nutritional risk.[148]

To chart your weight gain, use the grid on page 26. The numbers across the bottom line indicate the weeks of pregnancy; each number on the vertical line represents one pound of weight gained or lost.

Write your weight at conception in the space provided. Then each week place a dot to indicate your weight gain (or loss) since the last week. Every week weigh yourself on the same day (for example, every Tuesday), just after you get up in the morning and before you get dressed. Connect the dots to chart your rate of weight gain. The line on the chart represents a "typical" rate of weight gain.

### Baby-Building for the Normal-Weight Woman

A healthy, normal-weight woman should expect to gain 24 to 28 pounds during her pregnancy to produce a 7- to 8-pound baby, although the range might be even greater (20 to 35 pounds), given individual patterns.[146] Young women tend to gain more than older women; first-time mothers more than those who have had other children; thin women more than fat women.[132] The illustration on page 28 shows where the weight comes from.

Mary remembers, "One evening toward the end of my first pregnancy I was reading in bed and Peter, my husband, walked in. He stopped and looked at me and said, 'You look like a beached whale.' I felt like one too, despite the fact that I had gained a 'normal' 25 pounds. Short women can look *really* big. People asked me if I would deliver soon when I was in my sixth month!"

### Baby-Building for the Underweight Woman

The bad news is that, if you were very underweight prior to pregnancy and you gain less than 24 pounds during pregnancy, you are more likely to have a low-birth-weight child.

The good news is that, by gaining additional weight during

# CHART YOUR WEIGHT GAIN

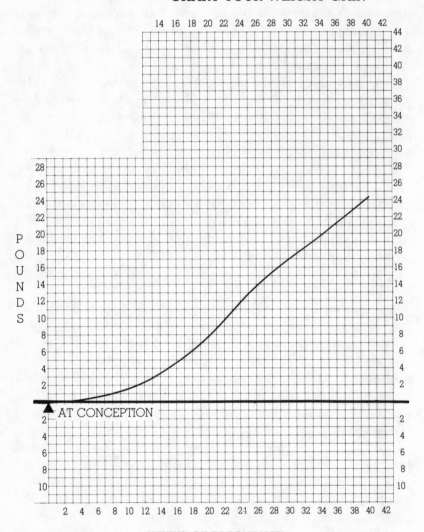

WEEKS OF PREGNANCY

pregnancy, you can reduce these risks. The optimal amount for you to gain would be 24 to 28 pounds *plus* the amount needed to bring you up to your ideal pre-pregnancy weight. For some women, this is simply not possible, but it is the goal.

If you have been underweight, your body is going to compete with your baby for nutrients. If the developing fetus does not get enough nutrients from the food you eat, it will draw upon your body. If your own stores are inadequate, your body will resist such deprivation. The woman who is underweight at the time she conceives and who does not gain normally during pregnancy risks developing toxemia, as described in Chapter 9. Your baby's needs will not be met, and your own health may be jeopardized.

The first thing you must do is determine *why* you are underweight. Do you like the way you look when you are thin? Is your weight the result of poor eating habits? Do you frequently skip meals or avoid whole categories of food? Are you a vegetarian? As you examine your reasons, rethink them in the light of your goal for pregnancy: a healthy baby.

The nutrition chapters in this book will be especially important for you to read because it is likely that you should improve your nutritional status. Your diet is vital to the normal development of your baby. It is hard to change established eating patterns, but it is only for a few months, and the effect will have lifetime implications for your child.

On the other hand, you may enjoy the added weight! As Sunni Reed noted: "At 5'8" and 117 pounds, I had for years been referred to as 'Gandhi' or as having that 'Care Package Look.' My gynecologist said, 'Eat what you like,' and I did. Fifty pounds later, I had breasts for the first time and an astounding belly, which from the rear was not noticeable but from the side reminded many people of a 'pregnant thermometer.' I was voluptuous for the only time in my life and loved it. I enjoyed the eating and delivered an eight-pound baby boy. Within six weeks, I returned to 117 pounds."

### Baby-Building for the Overweight Woman

This is not the time to concentrate on losing weight; it is the time to concentrate on growing a healthy baby. If you have had

# NORMAL WEIGHT GAIN IN PREGNANCY

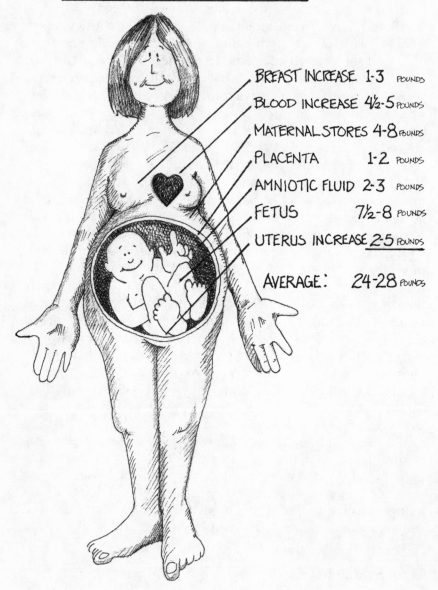

BREAST INCREASE 1-3 POUNDS

BLOOD INCREASE 4½-5 POUNDS

MATERNAL STORES 4-8 POUNDS

PLACENTA          1-2 POUNDS

AMNIOTIC FLUID 2-3 POUNDS

FETUS             7½-8 POUNDS

UTERUS INCREASE 2-5 POUNDS

AVERAGE:    24-28 POUNDS

trouble taking off pounds before you were pregnant, you will find it virtually impossible now. To begin with, your appetite may be "up" as Mother Nature tells you to feed the baby.

Some people assume that, if a woman is overweight, she is overnourished and probably has good nutrient stores. This simply is not true. There are many overweight women (and men too) whose diets are high in calories, sugar, and fat, but low in vital nutrients. It would be hard to find an obese person who gained the extra weight from excesses of fruits and vegetables, whole-grain breads, milk, and lean meats. Typically, the extra weight is from sugared or fried foods, alcohol, and snacks.

It has been said that obesity is the most prevalent form of malnutrition in the United States. The overweight woman needs to improve her diet during pregnancy at least as much as the underweight woman. *The emphasis must be on improving the* quality *of food choices so that nutrient needs will be met within a reasonable caloric intake.*

There are sound reasons why you should not diet during pregnancy. The growing fetus needs a steady, constant supply of nutrients and calories for optimal growth. If you skip meals or diet so that not enough calories are available from what you eat to meet the baby's need for energy, fat stores will be broken down within your body.

Broken-down fat cells are a poor source of energy for building a baby. When body fat is burned, it causes *ketones* (which are a form of acid) to be released. This can be detected in urine samples; your doctor may test for the presence of ketones if your rate of weight gain is not within a normal range. Ketones, especially if they occur during the last three months of pregnancy, can inhibit the development of your baby's brain. Cells do not develop normally in the acid environment created by the ketones.

The baby will, indeed, be drawing upon your reserves during its development, so your rate of weight gain and the total amount gained may be somewhat less than that of the normal-weight woman, usually in the range of 18 to 20 pounds.[52] According to *Nutrition & the M.D.*, "It is usually recommended that obese pregnant women gain approximately 24 pounds during gestation."[93]

The traditional reward of a slimmer figure that accompanies a successful weight-loss program just isn't going to happen during pregnancy. Go with the flow, and think about this as a period to concentrate on making every calorie count toward building that beautiful baby. You will be improving your eating habits during your pregnancy. The increased *quality* of your diet, as opposed to *quantity*, will help you shed pounds after delivery, especially if you decide to breastfeed. Work on a thinner you, *after* the baby is born and off to a good start in life.

### Is There Danger in Having a Big Baby?

We have made a case for establishing optimal birth weight at 7 pounds or more, but you may be wondering if there is a point at which a baby can be *too* big.

Few babies are born weighing over 9 or 9½ pounds. Babies this heavy are generally born to women with diabetes. It is very unlikely that you will have a baby this large as a result of excessive weight gain.

To set your mind at ease, you should know that large babies do not necessarily mean a long, arduous labor for the mother, or increased risk to the baby during delivery! This was a valid concern years ago, before obstetrical care had progressed to its current state.

There was a time when babies were delivered by Cesarean section only after hours of labor, when it became clear that the baby could not pass through the birth canal. Today, if the baby will not fit, usually it is known prior to or shortly after the onset of labor, and Cesarean section can alleviate a trying labor and difficult delivery.

Between 10 and 25 percent of all births in the United States are performed by Cesarean section today. By no means should the mother consider it a "failure" on her part.[149] It is a viable alternative that can avoid the need for a forceps delivery, which can potentially harm the child.

### Rate of Weight Gain

Many changes take place during the first few months of pregnancy. There are changes you can *feel*, but not necessarily *see.* Most women gain about 4 pounds in the first trimester. This is a physiological preparation in your body for the coming changes; at this point, the fetus weighs only a few ounces. Your weight gain at this time may be minimal, especially if you suffer from the nausea common to early pregnancy. While your weight may not be shooting up, you *will* notice changes in the shape of your body—goodbye waistline!

All of a sudden, usually at about the three-month mark, the baby really begins to shoot up (or out, we should say). From this point on, normal weight gain is about a pound a week, or a little less.

**PROCEED WITH CAUTION: CALL YOUR DOCTOR**

* If you suddenly gain
  2–5 pounds in one week
* If you gain less than
  2 pounds a month after
  your third month

### How Much Is Too Much?

Until recently, women were cautioned against gaining *too much* weight because they would get toxemia. The tide seems to have turned: now women are warned that if they do not gain *enough* weight, and eat a good diet, they will get (you guessed it) toxemia. A recent study of a large group of women who gained in excess of 30 pounds during pregnancy showed that while 9 percent developed toxemia, 91 percent did not.[132]

A report of the Committee on Maternal Nutrition of the National Research Council recommended that emphasis be placed on the value of the diet during pregnancy and advised against the restriction of the diet to lose weight.[158]

Although there is conflicting evidence about the dangers of excessive weight gain, there is considerable evidence to support the importance of adequate weight gain and the dangers of insufficient gain.[117] There is no accepted upper limit for "normal" weight gain because it is dependent upon weight at conception and many other factors. What used to be considered excessive is now thought to be normal. For our research, we did not find any medical authorities recommending a weight gain in excess of 35 pounds, for a woman entering pregnancy at desirable weight or above, and carrying a single child.

There are women who gain as much as 50 to 60 pounds, experience normal labor and delivery, and have healthy children. But the fewest risks and complications are associated with a weight gain within the recommended range.

If you gain excessively during the first two trimesters, you may be tempted to cut calories during the last three months. This is the time when your baby is growing the most. A weight-reduction plan will deprive your baby during a critical time. So try to plan ahead and pace your rate of weight gain, with some for you and some for baby.

Some common methods of weight control can be harmful when you are pregnant. If you find yourself eating too much and gaining too quickly, take the following steps:

---

## CUT CALORIES, BUT NOT NUTRIENTS

**Do:**
* Substitute skim, 1-percent or 2-percent milk for whole milk, but still drink four glasses a day.
* Omit all beverages that contain alcohol.
* Cut down on sources of sugar and fat.
* Avoid pastries, candy, soft drinks, rich desserts, snack foods; substitute fruit and fruit juices.
* Broil foods instead of frying.
* Use herbs and spices instead of rich sauces.
* Increase your physical activity.

**Do Not:**
* Skip meals.
* Cut out cereals or whole grains.
* Severely restrict salt.
* Use diuretics.

### Hello, Baby! Goodbye, Weight!

Your newborn baby will change your lifestyle and your body. In the week following their baby's birth, most women will lose the majority of the weight they gained during pregnancy. Another 4 to 6 pounds will be lost by the time the baby is six weeks old, and the remainder should disappear within three to six months. Be assured, women with normal weight gains during pregnancy rarely experience permanent weight gain. Anne remembers leaving the hospital in a trim shirtwaist dress with a belt after Lisa was born; Mary left still in maternity clothes—but both of us were at our regular weight a few months later.

Your body does need a few months to adjust the blood volume, body fluids, uterus size, and so on, but there is a way to expedite this process. Part of the "maternal reserve" that is gained during pregnancy is in preparation for breastfeeding. *Breastfeeding uses calories stored as pounds, and helps retract the uterus to its normal size.*

If you were underweight prior to pregnancy, you may look and feel better after adding a few pounds to your frame; if you are determined to return to your pre-pregnancy weight, resuming your pre-baby eating patterns will get you back to where you were.

The overweight or obese woman who has postponed dieting in the interest of her baby can now enter into a serious weight-loss program. Nursing your baby is a good kick-off to a goal of trimming excess pounds, although you will want to be sure that your diet is well-chosen so that you can produce enough milk. If you will be bottle-feeding, you will want to consider beginning a weight-reduction program based on sound nutrition principles. Regardless of how you will be feeding your baby, an exercise program will help you to both look and feel better.

# 3.
# The
# Nutritional
# Lifeline

From the moment of conception, the cells of the fetus need nutrients to survive. There must also be a means for eliminating waste materials that accumulate naturally. As embryonic cells divide and grow, a complex system evolves. About the third week of pregnancy, the fetal heart and bloodstream develop. From that point on, baby's blood and your blood do not mix. They exchange nutrients and waste materials through the *placenta. The placenta is the life-support system for the fetus.* It regulates the flow of oxygen and carbon dioxide, nutrients, and waste products, and produces at least six hormones that help sustain your pregnancy.[21]

The fetus is connected to the placenta by the *umbilical cord.* The cord contains one vein, which carries oxygen and nutrient-containing blood to the baby, and two arteries, which return waste products via the blood to the placenta. There are no nerves in the umbilical cord, which is why the baby feels no pain when the cord is cut at birth.[43] The umbilical vein and arteries project into the placenta in little rootlike structures called *villi.*

Your blood flows into the placenta where oxygen, nutrients, and some drugs and chemicals pass through the thin cellular walls of the villi and into the fetal circulatory system. This is the critical point where the transfer from mom to baby takes place. The placenta was once thought to act as a *barrier* to substances in the mother's blood that could harm the baby. Now we know that it blocks certain substances but not others. The size and other chemical features of substances in the blood determine whether the substances can cross the placenta. So it is more accurate to describe the placenta as a *filtering system* or *sieve*.

Many substances, such as glucose and sodium, go back and forth easily through the placenta, passing from the area where the substance is more concentrated to the area where the substance is less concentrated.

Unfortunately, many drugs, chemicals, and other substances that are potentially harmful can pass through the placenta filter as readily.

Most substances in the fetal bloodstream that are not used are carried back through the umbilical arteries, pass through the placenta, and return to the maternal bloodstream. Other substances, however, are converted in the fetus into complex forms or become trapped in the fetus and cannot pass back through the cell walls of the villi. Thus potentially harmful concentrations can build up in the fetus. Caffeine and vitamin C are examples of this one-way traffic that can cause problems if excessive amounts accumulate.

## Delivering Nutrients on Schedule

The average full-term pregnancy lasts 280 days, or approximately nine months. These nine months are divided into three trimesters. The baby grows and develops during all phases of pregnancy, but different parts of the body are developing at different times.

A good balanced diet with adequate calories, proteins, vitamins, and minerals helps your body support the pregnancy and contributes to the development and growth of your baby. Too many, or too few, nutrients, especially as organs are forming or bones or blood are building, can create fewer cells or ones that are less than perfectly formed.

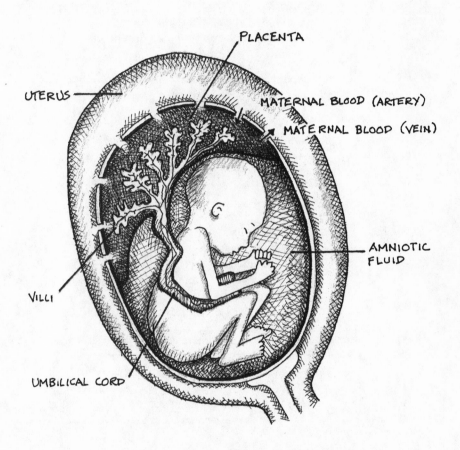

THE NUTRITIONAL LIFELINE

# YOUR BABY'S GROWTH

| Time | Development |
|------|-------------|
| **First Trimester:** | Vital need for good nutrition to support growth of maternal tissue and development of fetal internal organs, appendages, and sense organs. |
| Fertilization | |
| 7 days | Implantation in uterus |
| | Embryo is the size of the head of a pin |
| | Primitive circulation between placenta and embryo established |
| 4 weeks (1 month) | Beginning of eyes, ears, spine, digestive tract, limbs, nervous system, organs |
| | Heart begins functioning |
| 8 weeks (2 months) | Now called fetus |
| | Forming of hands and fingers |
| | Organs developing |
| | Heart beating |
| | Weight, about ⅓ ounce; about 1 inch long |
| 12 weeks (3 months) | Sex can be distinguished |
| | Tooth buds present |
| | Arms, hands, legs, feet, toes formed |
| | Moves in amniotic fluid (can't be felt by mother) |
| | Beginning of blood formation |
| | Weight, about 1 ounce; about 3 inches long |
| **Second Trimester:** | Crucial time for refinement of physical structure. |
| | Respiratory and cardiovascular systems are inadequately developed for life outside of mother's body. |
| | Mother's mineral intake important for developing strong bones and blood in fetus. |
| 16 weeks (4 months) | Scalp hair appears |
| | Motor activity begins |
| | Digestive system developed |
| | Heart muscle develops |
| | Kidneys in place |
| | Fetus now about 3–4 ounces; about 7 inches long |

| Time | Development |
|---|---|
| 20 weeks (5 months) | Legs lengthening<br>Calcification of baby teeth and long bones; flouride from fluoridated water now useful<br>Brain development continues<br>Usually baby's movements can be felt by mother<br>Fetus now about 10–11 ounces; 12 inches in length |
| 24 weeks (6 months) | Blood formation increases<br>Fatty protection of the nerve fiber begins; critical period of brain development<br>May be sucking thumb<br>Fetus usually about 1½–2 pounds; over a foot in length |
| **Third Trimester:** | Baby doubles in size in this trimester. Nutrients and calories are vital to development of the baby and for preservation of maternal stores. Transfer of minerals to baby's body to calcify bones and to build iron reserves in liver for the first few months of life. |
| 28 weeks (7 months) | Body developing fat<br>Nails appear<br>Lungs and eyes develop<br>Now about 3 pounds |
| 32 weeks (8 months) | Fetal weight increasing rapidly<br>Calcification of bones of fingers and toes<br>Teeth develop<br>Transfer of iron to baby's liver to protect against anemia in early infancy<br>Taste sense present<br>Developing reflexes and behavior patterns<br>Almost 4 pounds |
| 36 weeks (9 months) | Skin smooths as fat forms under it<br>Lungs fully developed<br>Metabolic system developing to support life after birth<br>Almost 5 pounds |
| 40 weeks (birth) | Skin smooth<br>Sex organs well developed<br>Insulation of brain begins; brain cells continue to develop<br>Able to sustain life outside womb<br>About 7+ pounds |

# 4.
# Major Nutrients: Protein, Carbohydrate, and Fat

## QUICK QUIZ

How much do you know about carbohydrate, protein, and fat? Answer these questions and then read the chapter. Correct answers are on page 233.

**True or False**

| | | |
|---|---|---|
| _F_ | 1. | Bran is the only source of fiber. |
| _F_ | 2. | Some peanut butter contains cholesterol. |
| _F_ | 3. | One gram of protein, one gram of carbohydrate, and one gram of fat each contain the same number of calories. |
| _T_ | 4. | Sucrose is another name for table sugar. |
| _F_ | 5. | Starches are more fattening than proteins. |
| _T_ | 6. | Pregnant women need more protein than most male athletes. |
| _F_ | 7. | Honey is a good source of many nutrients. |
| _T_ | 8. | Butter and margarine are equal in calories. |
| _T_ | 9. | Most Americans should include more starch in their diets. |
| _T_ | 10. | A low-carbohydrate diet is dangerous during pregnancy. |

41

Those who "speak nutrition" sometimes make it as difficult to understand as a foreign language. "Grams of protein" and "calories from carbohydrate" sound more like Greek than food. Just as the language course you take in a classroom doesn't really "take" until you find yourself in a situation where you need it in order to be understood, nutrition becomes much more meaningful when you see a reason for it. During pregnancy, every meal has an effect on you and on your baby.

What is nutrition? *Nutrition,* simply defined, is the process by which your body uses food. In the thousands of foods you eat or drink, there are only about fifty substances, or *nutrients,* that are absolutely essential. *These necessary nutrients can be categorized into six groups: protein, carbohydrate, fat, vitamins, minerals, and water.*

### Alphabet Soup

Throughout this book, there are many references to the RDAs. Sometimes we say "the RDA of the NRC." What is this? Who are they?

| | | |
|---|---|---|
| **RDA** | = | Recommended Dietary Allowances<br>The daily need for various nutrients. |
| **NRC** | = | National Research Council<br>The committee of experts who set the standards. |
| **U.S. RDA** | = | United States Recommended Dietary Allowances.<br>The RDA figures used on food labels by processors<br>who choose to provide nutritional information. |

The Recommended Dietary Allowances (RDAs) are goals for good nutrition which reflect current scientific thinking. Because of advances in knowledge, they are revised about every five years. The current RDAs, the Ninth Revised Edition, were published in 1980.[6] They include recommended levels of protein, calories, ten vitamins, and six minerals for daily consumption by healthy people. The table includes appropriate levels for pregnant women. The same committee estimated *ranges* of intake that they consider to be both safe and adequate for other vitamins and minerals about which less is known.

While there are U.S. RDAs specific to pregnant and lactating women, they are generally not those listed on labels except for prenatal vitamin-mineral supplements. The U.S. RDA percentages on most food labels are based on the needs of adults and children over 4 years of age. In this book, we refer to the *current RDA's* for pregnant and lactating women rather than the U.S. RDAs.

The U.S. RDAs listed on labels can help you identify good sources of particular nutrients. For example, a food that contains 30 percent of the daily U.S. RDA of a specific nutrient is a very good source, whether or not you are pregnant. If you see a food label with less than 5 percent of each nutrient, you know that this food does not contribute significantly to your diet.

The following chart will make you aware of your increased nutritional needs during pregnancy and lactation. In the following chapters, we will discuss the kinds of foods you can choose to meet these needs. *Nutrition is food, not numbers. You can eat well even if you do not understand the chart!*

## RECOMMENDED DIETARY ALLOWANCES FOR WOMEN [6]

|  | Female 19–22 yr. | Female 23–50 yr. | Pregnancy | Lactation** |
|---|---|---|---|---|
| Protein, grams | 44 | 44 | +30 | +20 |
| Vitamin A, retinol equivalents, micrograms | 800 | 800 | +200 | +400 |
| Vitamin D, micrograms | 7.5 | 5 | +5 | +5 |
| Vitamin E, alpha tocopherol equivalents, micrograms | 8 | 8 | +2 | +3 |
| Vitamin C, milligrams | 60 | 60 | +20 | +40 |
| Thiamin, milligrams | 1.1 | 1.0 | +0.4 | +0.5 |
| Riboflavin, milligrams | 1.3 | 1.2 | +0.3 | +0.5 |
| Niacin, niacin equivalents, milligrams | 14 | 13 | +2 | +5 |

## RECOMMENDED DIETARY ALLOWANCES
## FOR WOMEN [6] (cont.)

|  | Female 19–22 yr. | Female 23–50 yr. | Pregnancy | Lactation** |
|---|---|---|---|---|
| Vitamin B6, milligrams | 2.0 | 2.0 | +0.6 | +0.5 |
| Folacin, micrograms | 400 | 400 | +400 | +100 |
| Vitamin B12, micrograms | 3.0 | 3.0 | +1.0 | +1.0 |
| Calcium, milligrams | 800 | 800 | +400 | +400 |
| Phosphorus, milligrams | 800 | 800 | +400 | +400 |
| Magnesium, milligrams | 300 | 300 | +150 | +150 |
| Iron, milligrams | 18 | 18 | ** | *** |
| Zinc, milligrams | 15 | 15 | +5 | +10 |
| Iodine, micrograms | 150 | 150 | +25 | +50 |

*Lactation needs, where indicated by a +, are in addition to non-pregnant needs for age, *not* added to pregnancy needs.
**Increased need in excess of usually dietary intake; supplements of 30–60 mg. recommended.
***Continue supplementation for two to three months after delivery, then resume non-pregnancy level of intake.

## The Pro Team—Protein

Though a football coach may not agree, a pregnant woman needs proportionally more protein than his best quarterback! Contrary to popular belief, people engaged in sports and other strenuous activities do not need a significant increase in percentage of protein in their diets, if the total diet is otherwise adequate. Pregnant women, on the other hand, particularly sedentary ones, need extra protein for baby- and body-building.

Living things, large and small, are made of cells. Part of every cell is protein. Throughout life, protein must constantly be replenished to rebuild cells that are destroyed because of infection, surgery, or wear and tear. During pregnancy, when a whole new body is being constructed, protein is absolutely essential.

Protein builds bodies many ways. During pregnancy, protein helps build the tough fibrous tissue necessary for the baby's muscles, ligaments, hair, and fingernails, for the mother's uterus, and for the placenta. Protein helps build the baby's bones and teeth (even before birth). Protein is necessary for the transport of oxygen in the bloodstreams of both mother and baby—oxygen that is vital to the life of cells. The expanded volume of blood that is normal during pregnancy requires extra protein, too.

Protein plays a key role in regulating body processes. Body regulators have strange-sounding names, like *enzymes, hormones,* and *antibodies. Enzymes* initiate and promote chemical reactions in the body. Digestion, for example, requires a variety of enzymes to break down the food that we eat to nutrients that can be absorbed. *Hormones* have their ups and downs, especially during pregnancy. The hormones shift in balance to contribute to growth of the baby in addition to maintaining the mother's body. Some new hormones are manufactured by the placenta to regulate the way nutrients are used during pregnancy.[50] Adequate protein in the mother's diet permits the formation of these hormones. In addition, the baby begins producing hormones. Studies show that if mothers are severely deprived of protein during pregnancy, their babies may show abnormal growth patterns in early childhood because they have inadequate hormones.[169] *Antibodies* are the health protectors that ward off illness. What you eat today will not only help keep you healthy, but can help your child get a good start in life.

## All Protein Is Not of Equal Value

Proteins are made of *amino acids*. Different combinations of these components form different proteins. Protein in food or protein in body tissues can be broken down into individual amino acids, and then rearranged to make new proteins needed by your body or your baby's body. Like ingredients in recipes, they can be combined in different ways to make protein complexes needed for bones, brain tissue, blood, and the many other proteins needed for building and maintaining body cells.

The body manufactures most of the twenty-two amino acids

it needs, but there are nine it cannot produce. Since these nine must be supplied from foods you eat, they are called the *essential amino acids*. In order for your bundle of protein to grow, these nine *must* be present—*all* of them, and *at the same time*. You must be sure to eat foods that contain these important materials for your baby's growth.

| SOURCES OF PROTEIN | |
|---|---|
| 1. **Animal protein:** | meat, fish, poultry, eggs, dairy products (milk, cheese, yogurt) |
| 2. **Plant protein:** | grains (rice, corn, wheat); legumes (beans, soybeans); nuts and seeds (peanuts, sesame seeds, sunflower seeds); vegetables (green peas, broccoli); tofu (soybean curd) and other soy products |

Animal protein sources have some of each of the nine essential amino acids. They are called *complete proteins*. (An exception is gelatin. Though it comes from an animal source, it lacks an essential amino acid, and therefore cannot, by itself, build new cells for your fingernails or baby's tissues.)

Plant proteins contain most of the essential amino acids, but are low in or missing one or two of them. They are known as *incomplete proteins*. An incomplete protein cannot, by itself, build or repair tissues—it can only be used for energy. But by choosing several plant proteins at the same meal, you can supply all the essential nine ingredients for building tissues. *Vegetarians* and others who rely heavily on plant sources for food need to take care to eat protein foods that *complement* one another—such as beans with rice, cheese with noodles, peanut butter with whole-grain bread, and sesame seeds with garbanzo beans. The simple addition of milk to cereal gives the cereal grains body-building power.

There are many who practice vegetarianism in our country today. Some do so because of their religious beliefs; others abhor the thought of eating animals as food; still others do it because they feel it benefits their health or helps them control their weight. If you are a vegetarian, you may be very knowl-edgeable about mixing and matching to obtain the essential amino acids; but if you have been a "casual vegetarian," just skipping meats, your diet may not be good enough to meet the additional needs of pregnancy. Several excellent books that will help you understand the principles of choosing complementary proteins are listed on page 231.

If you eat no dairy products, such as cheese and milk, consult your doctor or a registered dietitian about the adequacy of your diet for pregnancy. Chances are, you will have to have a tailormade plan to meet your needs for protein, calcium, and other nutrients essential to make a healthy baby.

Many women today choose diets that exclude red meat. They can get ample protein from eggs, fish, poultry, dairy products, and a variety of foods from plant sources to meet their protein needs during pregnancy.

Animal studies show that nature has devised a way of partially protecting the fetus's needs for protein. If the mother's diet is deficient in protein, her own tissues will be broken down to provide some of the protein necessary for the baby's development. Some studies have suggested that toxemia, (discussed in Chapter 9) is related to consumption of a diet low in protein.

In this country, most women have diets that are adequate in protein. There is little danger of mother or baby being deprived of this nutrient. In fact, most pregnant women get more than enough protein. You do not need to be concerned if you follow the suggestions in Chapter 7.

When severe undernutrition takes place, both physical and mental growth of the baby can be restricted.[14] The baby's brain is developing throughout pregnancy, but during a series of critical days near the end of pregnancy, brain cells multiply at a very rapid rate. If adequate protein is not available, fewer cells form. This is a situation that may permanently limit physical and mental development.

### How Much Protein Is Needed?

During the first weeks, you might think that there would be no need for additional protein because your baby isn't even as big as a peanut yet. But important changes that require protein are taking place in your body. The placenta is developing; your uterus is changing; amniotic fluid is forming; blood volume is increasing; breast tissue is growing. In addition, your body begins to build stores for the times ahead that will demand a steady flow of protein to meet the needs of rapid fetal growth. All this may happen before you are even sure that you are pregnant!

For healthy women the NRC recommends increasing protein intake by 30 grams a day, from the beginning of pregnancy. This is in addition to the 45 to 50 grams needed by non-pregnant women. Therefore, you now need 75 to 80 grams of protein daily. Adolescents and women who are underweight may need even more.[6] In order to meet these needs, you must be able to translate grams of protein into food choices. Use the chart below.

For protein to do its job of tissue building, adequate *calories* must be consumed. If you eat lots of protein but insufficient calories, you will burn the protein for energy and it will not be used for building tissue.

The body is selective about its sources of calories. The primary source is carbohydrate. If carbohydrate becomes depleted, fat is used. If both fat and carbohydrate are inadequate for energy needs, protein will be diverted away from its tissue-building and regulating functions to be used for energy. *Some protein can be converted to carbohydrate and fat, but nothing can do the job of protein except protein.* This is why, during pregnancy, you will want to have enough calories from carbohydrates and fat to "spare the protein."

## Carbohydrates—The Fuel of Human Life

Carbohydrates have received an undeserved bad reputation over the years. It is now recommended that we increase our consumption of carbohydrates from fresh fruits and vegetables and whole grains.

Restricting carbohydrates can be very dangerous, especially during pregnancy. A number of popular diets, including the Atkins, Stillman, and Scarsdale diets, are based on eating fewer

## PROTEIN IN FOOD [34]

Need in Pregnancy—About 75 to 80 Grams of Protein Daily

|  | Portion | Grams of Protein |
|---|---|---|
| Tuna, oil packed, drained | ½ cup | 28 |
| Chicken, broiled, without skin | 3½ oz. | 24 |
| Beef: lean sirloin | 3 oz. | 24 |
| hamburger | 1 medium | 22 |
| Chili, beef and beans | 1 cup | 23 |
| Fish, broiled | 3½ oz. | 21 |
| Cottage cheese | 3½ oz. | 14 |
| Taco | 1 medium | 12 |
| Chick peas (garbanzos) | 3½ oz. | 10 |
| Peanut butter | 2 Tbsp. | 8 |
| Milk—skim, 1%, 2%, whole | 1 cup | 8 |
| Cheese: American, Cheddar, Gouda, Muenster, Swiss | 1 oz. | 7 |
| Bologna | 2 oz. | 7 |
| Egg, boiled | 1 medium | 6 |
| Soup: split pea | 1 cup | 7 |
| chicken noodle | 1 cup | 5 |
| cream of mushroom | 1 cup | 2 |
| Oatmeal | 1 cup | 5 |
| Potato, baked | 1 medium | 4 |
| Broccoli, cooked | 1 large stalk | 3 |
| Nuts, mixed | 8–12 | 3 |
| Ice cream | ½ cup | 3 |
| Bread: white, whole wheat, rye, raisin, Italian | 1 slice | 2 |
| Rice | ½ cup | 2 |
| Cornflakes | 1 cup | 2 |
| Carrots, raw | 2 small | 1 |

carbohydrates. The theory is that if you deprive the body of carbohydrates, excess body fat will be burned for fuel.

A low-carbohydrate diet is a serious threat to an unborn child. *The baby must have a constant supply of fuel from carbohydrates for development of the brain and nervous system.* Damage can occur if there is deprivation of carbohydrate for even a short period of time. Dr. Atkins is quoted as saying, "I'm sorry . . . I recommended the diet during pregnancy. I now understand that [it] could result in fetal damage."[19]

The idea of limiting carbohydrate consumption would be unthinkable to most of the world's population, many of whom derive 80 percent of their food energy from carbohydrate-rich foods such as rice, beans, wheat, and corn. In the United States and Canada, where carbohydrates provide only 40 to 50 percent of food energy, there is potential danger of underestimating their value in the total diet.

We have established the importance of sparing protein calories for baby building. Where do the calories come from? Fat has calories that can be used for energy, but medical researchers are now telling us that we should cut down the amount of fat in our diets. Calories from fat cannot be used efficiently by the brain and nervous system. We don't advise alcohol as a source of calories, especially during pregnancy. The only remaining source of calories is carbohydrates. It is also the best fuel for body energy. *Usually abundant and relatively inexpensive, carbohydrate-rich foods, derived primarily from plants, are the fuel of human life.*

### The Making of a Carbohydrate

This next section is going to get technical, but if you can follow along, it will not only help you understand *why* you should eat carbohydrates, but it will prepare you for the inevitable day when your child wants you to help with a homework assignment about photosynthesis.

Unlike plants, humans cannot synthesize nutrients from sunlight; we need to use plants as intermediaries. Here is how this happens:

Some of the energy the sun gives to plants is trapped within the plant and stored as glucose, a form of carbohydrate. (Like solar-heated water, stored in tanks.) When the plant is eaten, digestive enzymes dissolve the bonds holding the glucose and the plant energy is released to provide human energy (as the hot water is released to heat your home).

Because of its chemical structure, *glucose* is classified as a "simple" carbohydrate or simple sugar. Sometimes the atoms of glucose are rearranged to become other forms of simple sugars called fructose and galactose. These are found in fruits such as bananas, cherries, and berries, and in honey.

The scientific word for sugar is *saccharide*. Simple sugars are called *monosaccharides*. Two simple sugars can be joined together to form "double sugars." Double sugars are called *disaccharides*. Maltose is a combination of two glucose units; lactose, found in milk, is a combination of the simple sugars galactose and glucose. If fructose and glucose are bonded together, they form *sucrose*. Sucrose on your breakfast table is known as sugar. It is derived primarily from sugar cane or sugar beets.

As plants mature, they build up stores of excess energy in seeds. Since glucose is not stable enough to endure this storage process, it is transformed into a more durable form. The stored glucose is called *starch*. Going back to our analogy, starch would be a solar-energy battery. Where the sugars are identified as "simple" carbohydrates, starch is classified as a "complex" carbohydrate, chemically a *polysaccharide*. Plant starch is a major source of carbohydrate in our diets. It is available in plant seeds such as potatoes, corn, and rice. Because starch molecules are encased in a tough skin, we usually cook starch-containing foods before we eat them to soften the cell walls. Our bodies cannot absorb starch, so the process of digestion is used to break down the starch into basic glucose units to meet energy needs.

Some of the units of glucose in the plant stems, leaves, bark, roots, and seeds are linked together in such a way that they cannot be broken down by human enzymes. These glucose chains are called *cellulose*. Cellulose, because it is not digested and absorbed, provides no calories, but it is a source of *fiber* or *roughage* in our diets. *Pectins* and *gums* are other polysaccharides that are soft and "sticky" forms of fiber. Fiber passes through the digestive tract and into the intestines with relatively little breakdown. Along the way, fiber absorbs water and swells to give a sensation of fullness. The pregnant woman who finds herself with an insatiable appetite may find some satisfaction from these foods. Celery, carrots, and green peppers are good choices of high-fiber/low-calorie foods. Other good sources of dietary fiber, such as raisins, dried apricots, nuts, and seeds, contain more calories, along with vitamins and minerals.

Fiber is especially important during pregnancy because it helps prevent constipation and hemorrhoids. Fruits, vegetables, and grains contain different forms of fiber, each of which can be useful in keeping your body running smoothly. Dried and raw fruits and raw vegetables usually have more fiber than cooked or canned ones because the heating process breaks down some of the fiber.

*Bran* is the most publicized form of fiber, but recent evidence suggests that softer fiber in fruits and vegetables may have a more positive effect.[175] Too much bran or other fiber, when added to foods, can prevent the absorption of some vitamins and minerals.

If your diet contains few of these foods, we suggest you

## GOOD SOURCES OF DIETARY FIBER

| Bread | Vegetables | Fruits |
|---|---|---|
| Cornbread | All raw vegetables | Apples with skin |
| Cracked-wheat bread | Brussels sprouts | Berries |
| Crackers with seeds | Cabbage | Dired apricots |
| Dark breads (e.g. pumpernickel) | Corn | Pears with skin |
| Rye | Parsnips | Prunes |
| Rye crisp | Peas | Raisins |
| Whole-grain crackers | | |
| Whole wheat | *Nuts and Seeds* | |
| | All | |
| *Grains* | *Legumes* | *Cereals* |
| Brown rice | Baked beans | Bran |
| Buckwheat groats | Black-eyed peas | Grape-Nuts |
| Bulgur | Chick peas (garbanzos) | Oatmeal |
| Popcorn | Kidney beans | Shredded wheat |
| Wheat germ | Lima beans | |

increase them moderately at first, and let your system adjust gradually to the increase in fiber. Drink plenty of liquids to replace the water from your body that is absorbed by fiber as it passes through.

### Natural vs. Refined Carbohydrates

We have identified three types of carbohydrates: sugars, starch, and cellulose (fiber). But there is another distinction to be made. There are naturally available carbohydrates and there are refined or processed carbohydrates. The *naturally available carbohydrates* are in foods as they grow. Not only are they a source of energy, at the rate of four calories per gram, they are generally accompanied by a variety of other nutrients such as vitamins and minerals. Fruits, vegetables, and grains contain natural carbohydrates.

*Refined or processed carbohydrates* are extracted from natural sources, such as sugarcane or sugar beets, and may be added to foods. Sugar has a legitimate role in food processing. It can increase palatability, make foods brown evenly during baking, and contribute to texture. On the other hand, some highly sweetened processed foods contribute little more than calories to your diet. Many that are high in refined sugar content, such as soda pop, candy, cookies, and pastries, are woefully devoid of vitamins and minerals.

To many people, "sugar" means table sugar, or sucrose. Yet this is only one of a large group of sweeteners found in foods.

When you read a food label, look at the ingredient list to find out if sweeteners have been added. If any of the sweeteners listed is first on the ingredient list, you know that there is more sweetener than anything else in the food! Many foods contain several of these ingredients, but they all serve the same purpose—to sweeten your food.

Some believe that white sugar is bad for you and that *honey* and *raw sugar* are healthier. Neither of these beliefs is true. The basic difference is in flavor rather than nutritional value. True raw sugar is not marketed in the United States because it is too impure and poses a potential health hazard. What is referred to as "raw sugar" is turbinado sugar. *Turbinado sugar* is purified like refined white sugar, but not all of the molasses has been removed. The molasses contains small amounts of iron and B vitamins. Honey, a combination of glucose and fructose, has traces of a few vitamins and minerals. Given the small amount of turbinado sugar or honey we eat, little can be said for either as a source of nutrients. Honey is an expensive source of calories. If you like the taste of honey, enjoy it, but don't believe that it has particular health benefits.

## SWEETENERS

| | | |
|---|---|---|
| Brown sugar | High fructose | Powdered sugar |
| Carob powder |   corn syrup | Saccharin |
| Confectioners' | Honey | Sorbitol |
|   sugar | Invert sugar | Sorghum |
| Corn syrup | Maltose | Sucrose, table |
| Cyclamates | Mannitol |   sugar |
| Dextrin | Mannose | Turbinado sugar |
| Dextrose | Maple syrup | Xylitol |
| Fructose |   or Maple sugar | |
| Glucose | | |

## NUTRIENTS IN SUGAR AND HONEY [34]

| Portion | Calories | Carbo-hydrate (gm) | Protein (gm) | Calcium (mg) | Iron (mg) | Thiamin (mg) | Vit. C (mg) |
|---|---|---|---|---|---|---|---|
| Sugar (1 Tbsp.) | 46 | 11.9 | 0 | trace | 0 | 0 | 0 |
| Honey (1 Tbsp.) | 61 | 16.5 | 0.1 | 1 | 0.1 | 0 | trace |

### The Role of Carbohydrates During Pregnancy

Your body runs twenty-four hours a day and needs a continuous supply of fuel to keep it going. Even when you're sleeping, your heart continues to beat, you continue to breathe, digestion continues, and the basic tasks of maintaining your body go on. In addition, during pregnancy, your baby is on a round-the-clock growing program that burns up energy at about twice the rate your own body does.

Carbohydrates are the major source of body fuel. The carbohydrates that you consume in food are converted by digestion into glucose, which is then quickly absorbed into the bloodstream and soon is on the way to performing its many tasks.

Fortunately, we don't have to eat constantly to provide the steady flow of energy that is required. Simple-sugar carbohydrates are converted to glucose very rapidly, and can be used to meet immediate energy needs. The more complex starches take longer to be broken down, and therefore provide energy over a longer period of time. Some glucose can be stored in the liver. To do this it must be converted to *glycogen*, the body's form of starch. But just so much glycogen can be stored—usually enough to last overnight.

### How Much Carbohydrate Is Enough?

How much carbohydrate does it take during pregnancy to maintain energy needs and spare protein? Generally, about half of the total calories you consume should come from carbohydrates, especially the naturally occurring ones, which come packaged with other nutrients. Whole grains and fresh fruit and vegetables, for instance, are high in fiber and low in fat, refined sugar, and salt—and they are rich in vitamins and minerals. Skim or lowfat milk is also a valuable source of carbohydrates, protein, vitamins, and minerals. The Nutritional Game Plan, Chapter 7, is a balanced plan that provides all the essential nutrients for a healthy pregnancy; it guides you in selecting the best carbohydrates. Carbohydrates are nature's bargain nutrients. In order to get your money's worth, choose carbohydrates that give you the extras along with the calories.

### Fats: The Protectors

At the beginning of this chapter, we identified the essential nutrients: protein, carbohydrates, fat, vitamins, minerals, and water. The least essential is fat.

Dietary fats add flavor, texture, and odor to foods. We look for well-marbled meat. We add butter to our baked potato for flavor. The smell of bacon cooking makes our mouths water. A little bit of butter makes many foods more palatable. We enjoy dressings on our salads.

Because fats tend to stay in the stomach a bit longer than carbohydrates and proteins, they are more satisfying. This phenomenon gives a sense of fullness.

Some essential nutrients are found only in fat-containing foods: vitamins A, D, E, and K, and linoleic acid. If the fat is removed from a food, as it is in skim milk, these vitamins are also removed. Vitamins A and D are added back to skim milk through the process of fortification.

Fat contains *linoleic acid*, essential for the development of brain cells and the central nervous system of your baby. Linoleic acid cannot be produced by the body. The need for a dietary source was established when premature babies fed nonfat formulas developed severe skin problems.

Before you run out to buy linoleic-acid supplements, we must say that there is virtually no danger of a deficiency. Most adult women, even those who eat as little as two tablespoons of fat in a whole day, get enough linoleic acid to meet their own needs and needs imposed during pregnancy.

Gram for gram (a gram is a bit less than a quarter-teaspoon), *you get more than twice as many calories in fat as in carbohydrate or protein*. Fat provides nine calories of energy for every gram, compared to four calories in each gram of carbo-hydrate or protein. Some of these calories help meet immediate energy needs; others will be stored as energy reserves. A limited amount of carbohydrate is stored as glycogen in the liver (this only lasts about ten hours); surplus protein, carbohy-drate, and fat are all converted to the fat bank for use as emergency energy reserves. Many of us would like a little less fat in our bank!

As pregnancy progresses, fat stores help meet the increas-ing energy demands of rapid fetal growth. The added weight and bulk created by fat reserves may be difficult for you to accept, but it is Nature's way of protecting the baby in the critical period before birth, during labor and delivery, and during breastfeeding. Fat in your breasts protects the mammary glands; a pad of fat under kidneys cushions them when you walk or jog and protects them if you should fall; a layer of insulating fat under your skin keeps you and your baby warm in cold weather.

When fat is burned in the absence of carbohydrates, the result is a condition known as *ketosis,* a high concentration of acid in the blood. Even a mild case of ketosis can be dangerous during pregnancy. Growing cells do not develop very well in this acid environment, and brain cells seem to be especially vulnerable.[172] So skipping meals during the last trimester to limit weight gain can have consequences other than weight control. Your doctor may test your urine for the presence of ketones and may tell you to add carbohydrate if ketones are present.

We've established the role of fat in maintaining health and promoting maximum well-being of the fetus. Too much of this good thing, however, has the fat deposits of many Americans bulging. We must emphasize once more that *pregnancy is no time to diet,* but it is a time when you should improve your eating habits and reduce consumption of calorie-packed fat-rich foods, and concentrated sweets.

Many fats in foods are hidden. Few people realize, for example, that most cold cuts and many cheeses have more fat than protein. One slice (1 ounce) of American cheese has twice the fat as a half cup of creamed cottage cheese. Isn't it ironic that creamed cottage cheese is a really lowfat food? Many foods contain fat, but lots of extra fat and calories are added by the cook!

### Types of Fat

The protein qualifiers are *complete* and *incomplete*; the carbohydrates are divided into *sugars, starches,* and *fiber.* Fat is categorized as *saturated, unsaturated,* and *polyunsaturated.*

All food fats, whether animal or vegetable in origin, contain a mixture of saturated and unsaturated fats. Usually, animal fats are more saturated and vegetable fats are primarily unsaturated. Some animals contain greater percentages of saturated fats than others; some vegetable fats are more unsaturated than others. Generally, the more solid a fat is, the

## FATS IN FOOD [34]

| Food | Portion Size | Grams of Fat[*] |
|---|---|---|
| Bologna | 2 oz. | 16 |
| Avocado | ½ medium | 16 |
| Beef: hamburger | 1 medium | 15 |
|     lean sirloin | 3 oz. | 7 |
| Oils: corn, safflower, peanut | 1 Tbsp. | 14 |
| Bacon, crisp | 3 strips | 14 |
| Sweet roll | 1 medium | 14 |
| Soup: cream of mushroom | 1 serving | 11 |
|     chicken noodle | 1 serving | 1 |
| French fries | small serving | 10 |
| Corn chips | 1 oz. | 10 |
| Frankfurter | 1 medium | 10 |
| Chocolate bar | 1 oz. | 10 |
| Cream cheese | 2 Tbsp. | 10 |
| Nuts, mixed | 8–12 | 9 |
| Ham | 3 oz. | 9 |
| French dressing | 1 Tbsp. | 9 |
| Milk | | |
|     whole | 1 cup | 9 |
|     2% | 1 cup | 5 |
|     1% | 1 cup | 3 |
|     skim | 1 cup | 0 |
| Ice cream | ½ cup | 8 |
| Cheese: American, Swiss, | | |
|     Muenster, Gouda | 1 oz. | 8 |
| Peanut butter | 2 Tbsp. | 8 |
| Tuna, oil-packed, drained | ½ cup | 8 |
|     water-packed | ½ cup | 1 |
| Fish, broiled | 3½ oz. | 7 |
| Sour cream | 2 Tbsp. | 6 |
| Mayonnaise | 1 Tbsp. | 6 |
| Egg, boiled | 1 medium | 6 |
| Creamed cottage cheese | 3½ oz. | 4 |
| Chicken, broiled, without skin | 3½ oz. | 4 |
| Most fruits and vegetables | 1 serving | 0 |

[*]One gram of fat has 9 calories. Most of these foods also have calories from protein and/or carbohydrate.

more saturated it is; liquid fats (oils) are the most unsaturated and are called polyunsaturated. Vegetable oil that has been processed to become margarine is partially saturated to make it solid.

### The Cholesterol Controversy

The Dietary Guidelines for the United States include one that reads, *"Avoid too much fat, saturated fat, and cholesterol."*[162]

Many saturated fats also contain cholesterol—a much-discussed fatlike substance. *Cholesterol* is a form of fat produced only in animals, including humans. It is never found in plants.

Many (including the American Heart Association) believe that the general public should eat less cholesterol-rich foods, while others believe that only those with documented high-cholesterol levels should decrease consumption. There are many variables including the amount of cholesterol your body itself produces. Most of us produce (in our bodies) far more cholesterol than we eat. Your body's predisposition to retain cholesterol is influenced by genetics. These factors cannot be readily controlled, but additional cholesterol from dietary sources can be limited by food choices.

Whether to suggest that the general public limit cholesterol is one of the great current nutrition debates. Much of the research on cholesterol was done on middle-aged males. There are fewer data on younger populations and no evidence that cholesterol is harmful during pregnancy. Studies of cholesterol done on pregnant women are inconclusive. Because of the profound physiological changes that occur during pregnancy, pregnant women cannot be judged by the standards of non-pregnant women. Cholesterol may be needed because of an increase in hormone levels and for the formation of your baby's brain tissue, so some elevation in your blood is to be expected.

*Unless your doctor, as a result of blood tests, finds a demonstrated reason for you to avoid cholesterol, you need not be cautious about dietary cholesterol during pregnancy.*

Liver is a food high in cholesterol, but since it is not consumed daily, and is not incorporated into other foods, do not use its cholesterol content as an excuse to avoid eating it. Egg yolks are the major contributor to your daily intake of

cholesterol. Both liver and eggs contain a variety of nutrients
and are excellent sources of protein, so they should be included
in your diet while you are pregnant. There is no essential need
for foods containing cholesterol; your body can manufacture
all the cholesterol you'll need before, during and after pregnancy. If you are preparing meals for your family, especially
men and boys, limiting foods rich in cholesterol may be the
prudent course.

## Nine Months and Seventy-five Thousand Calories Later

It takes roughly seventy-five thousand calories, in addition
to your own need for calories, to make a baby. Providing these
calories is the first nutritional requirement of pregnancy. A
healthy combination of calories for your pregnancy menu
would look something like the following illustration.

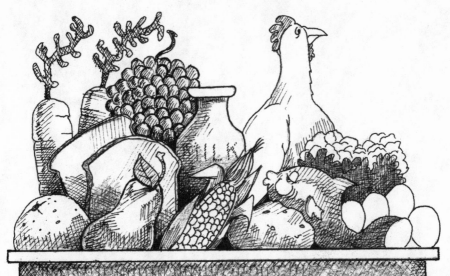

10% REFINED SUGAR

55% CARBOHYDRATES

45% STARCHES AND
NATURALLY OCCURRING SUGARS

10% POLYUNSATURATED
10% UNSATURATED
10% SATURATED

30% FATS

## THE FOOD BOWL

# 5.
# Vitamins:
# Small but Mighty

## QUICK QUIZ

How much do you know about vitamins? Choose the one correct response. Answers are on page 233.

1. The best source of Vitamin C among the following foods is:
   - **a.** a slice of bread
   - **b.** a glass of milk
   - **c.** a beef patty
   - **d.** a green pepper

2. The vitamin formed by the action of sunlight on the skin is:
   - **a.** Vitamin A
   - **b.** Vitamin C
   - **c.** Vitamin D
   - **d.** Niacin

3. If you have been taking birth-control pills, you probably need additional amounts of:
   - **a.** Vitamin A
   - **b.** Vitamin E
   - **c.** Vitamin D
   - **d.** Vitamin $B_6$

4. Large doses of which vitamin have been found to be particularly dangerous?
   - **a.** Vitamin A
   - **b.** Thiamin
   - **c.** Vitamin $B_{12}$
   - **d.** Niacin

5. The vitamin needed especially by pregnant women and when cells are dividing or growing is:
   - **a.** Thiamin
   - **b.** Folacin
   - **c.** Vitamin $B_{12}$
   - **d.** Vitamin A

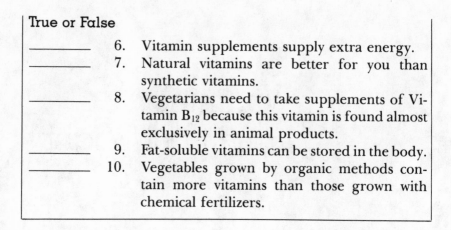

**True or False**

_____ 6. Vitamin supplements supply extra energy.
_____ 7. Natural vitamins are better for you than synthetic vitamins.
_____ 8. Vegetarians need to take supplements of Vitamin $B_{12}$ because this vitamin is found almost exclusively in animal products.
_____ 9. Fat-soluble vitamins can be stored in the body.
_____ 10. Vegetables grown by organic methods contain more vitamins than those grown with chemical fertilizers.

Remember the old word-association game? The one where I say a word and you respond immediately with whatever comes to mind? If I say "nutrition," there's a good chance your response would be "vitamins."

It's no wonder! Many of us have been raised by mothers who implored us, "Take your vitamins, so you'll grow up to be strong and healthy." We want no less for our children.

All the vitamins you need in a whole day amount to about an eighth of a teaspoon! But quantity is no indication of importance in this case. _Vitamins are essential for life and growth._ They have been called the "spark plugs" of life because all the body processes depend directly or indirectly on them. One of the first things your doctor may do when he finds you are pregnant is prescribe vitamin supplements. This raises questions.

**Question: If I do not have time for breakfast or lunch, will an extra vitamin pill do?**
Answer: No. Vitamins cannot replace food. Using the analogy of vitamins being like spark plugs, we might say that you cannot run a car or a body on spark-plug power alone. You need fuel and raw materials from carbohydrates, protein, and fat in foods.

**Question: Will vitamin supplements give me energy when I feel tired?**

Answer: If you think that vitamin supplements provide energy, you are in good company. A recent survey showed that 75 percent of all Americans believe this.[66] It is *not* true! Energy comes from calories, and *vitamins contain no calories.* What *is* true is that if you happen to be deficient in one of the vitamins necessary to *release* energy from glucose (thiamin, for example), you will be tired, and replacement of the missing nutrient will alleviate the symptom.

**Question: Are "natural" vitamin supplements better than "synthetic" vitamin supplements?**

Answer: Vitamins rate right up there with the American flag and apple pie when it comes to truth and goodness. It comes as a shock to find that *all vitamins are chemicals.*

Each vitamin has a specific chemical structure, and these chemical configurations can be duplicated by chemists in laboratories. In order to be vitamin C, the molecules must be arranged in a specific pattern; otherwise, a compound is not vitamin C. So vitamin C is vitamin C, whether it is found in an orange or in a capsule.

Claims have been made that natural vitamin supplements are less likely to cause allergic reactions than synthetic ones, but there are no clinical data to support this. Your body cannot tell whether the vitamin supplement you consume comes from a natural source or a chemical laboratory.

Consumers Union reported that because making vitamins from natural sources (fruits, for example) is an expensive process, some "natural" vitamins are made with added chemically formulated vitamins.[7] *Natural vitamin supplements are no better, nor worse, than synthetic ones; they are more expensive.*

**Question: Do organically grown foods contain more vitamins than foods grown "commercially"?**

Answer: There is a widespread belief that foods available in the neighborhood supermarket do not contain adequate vitamins because modern farming techniques have depleted the soil and reduced the nutrient content of fruits and vegetables grown there. The nutrient content of food is the same, whether they are grown in rich or poor soil. A carrot may be smaller if grown in poor soil, or the crop may be meager, but it is still a standard source of nutrients. When carrots from various sources are tested in laboratories, using the latest technology, it cannot be determined which carrots were grown by "commercial" or "organic, natural" methods. There are many studies which show that nutrient value and amounts of chemical residues are comparable.[8]

More is known about agricultural techniques for optimal production than ever before; a greater variety of fresh and frozen vegetables and fruits is available today because of sophisticated harvesting and distribution systems. In the often-longed-for "good old days," there were limited supplies of a few fruits and vegetables that happened to be in season—and their quality depended on weather and other environmental conditions. For some people, this modern technology has brought great anxiety and fear; but for the majority of consumers in our country, it has brought a variety of wholesome, economical foods that would otherwise be unattainable.

### Question: Will "extra" vitamins during pregnancy make me and my baby healthier?

Answer: There are two schools of thought about what vitamins do. Some people believe that huge quantities of vitamin supplements can prevent and cure diseases; others say adequate vitamins are available in foods and supplements should be taken only if deficiencies exist, and to treat a few disorders specifically related to vitamin imbalances. Vitamins were virtually unknown until the twentieth century. Vitamin research has only just begun. What some would take to be inconclusive test results, others assume to be sure evidence of positive needs. Active Americans love vitamin pills because they offer quick and easy solutions to complex problems—fast-food health! Not surprisingly, those who profit from the sale of millions of dollars of vitamin pills annually are active proponents of vitamin supplements as solutions to virtually all medical and emotional problems.

**Question: Can vitamins be dangerous?**

Answer: Excessive amounts of vitamins (*megadoses*) can be very dangerous to both you and your baby during pregnancy. Your baby can "overdose" if large amounts of some vitamins become highly concentrated in the fetal bloodstream. The baby can build up a vitamin tolerance that can result in his suffering withdrawal symptoms when levels are reduced after birth. If you are taking large amounts of vitamin supplements, or are considering doing so during your pregnancy, you may be jeopardizing the health and well-being of your child. *Do not risk exposing your baby to uncertain vitamin therapies that are potentially harmful.*

Large doses of vitamins may be indicated in cases verified by abnormally low blood levels of specific nutrients, and then they should be taken only under medical supervision. Vitamins prescribed for therapeutic reasons are not considered nutrients, but drugs.

Mary's brother, Fred (now an international lawyer, who will surely be humiliated by the story), spent his undergraduate years at the University of California at Berkeley. While there, he was "into" fruits and nuts and, during one period, was existing on carrot juice as a major part of his diet. Carrot juice is an excellent source of carotene, the vegetable form of vitamin A, which is also an orange pigment.

As Mary remembers, "Fred appeared at my door one evening after driving across the country. He was a nice shade of *peach*! At first I thought he had jaundice, until I looked more carefully. He had a curious problem called *xanthosis cutis*, which occurs when fat-containing cells pick up carotene pigment. He had not even noticed it because he had 'oranged' gradually. I evaluated his diet and he gave up his juices and returned to a more normal and varied eating pattern. It took about a month for Fred to fade."

This can also happen to infants who are given too many orange, deep yellow, or green baby foods. It does no permanent damage, but it is close to overdosing on food! *Toxicity is unlikely if you get your vitamins from foods.*

**Question: Does every woman need vitamin supplements during pregnancy?**

Answer: The question must be answered on an individual basis, depending on specific needs identified by your doctor. If you are a vegetarian, for instance, special supplements may be needed. If you have been on "the Pill" until just before becoming pregnant, your vitamin needs may require special supplements.

If you are healthy and eat a well-balanced diet, vitamin supplements may not be necessary, but most doctors prescribe a prenatal vitamin-mineral supplement as a "nutrition insurance policy," to be used in concert with a good diet. *Prenatal vitamin supplements are formulated to be balanced and emphasize the nutrients you and your baby need.*

Most prenatal supplements are a combination of vitamins and minerals. All include the mineral iron, and folic acid, a vitamin. Vitamin $B_{12}$ supplements are needed for women eating vegetarian diets that exclude all animal products.[151A]

## Thirteen Vital Vitamins

Contrary to reports in some nonprofessional nutrition publications, and labels that appear on the myriad number of vitamins being offered for sale, there are only thirteen vitamins known to be essential for health.

1. Vitamin A
2. Thiamin
3. Riboflavin
4. Niacin
5. Vitamin $B_6$
6. Vitamin $B_{12}$
7. Folacin
8. Pantothenic Acid
9. Biotin
10. Vitamin C
11. Vitamin D
12. Vitamin E
13. Vitamin K

Also called
"The B Vitamins"

## What You Need to Know About Vitamins

Do not be overwhelmed by the charts that follow! We have highlighted points that are especially important for you to know about during your pregnancy. The information is organized to be used as a reference when you have specific questions about vitamins.

■ *Category:* A vitamin is known by the way it is absorbed and stored. . . . Vitamins are classified as *fat-soluble* or *water-soluble*. While water-soluble vitamins must be provided each day from foods, the fat-soluble vitamins can be stored in our bodies.

■ *Other Names:* A vitamin by any other name . . . By becoming familiar with the varied terminology used to identify vitamins, you can begin to sort fact from fiction. For instance, if you read about the wonders of pyridoxine, you will find that pyridoxine is just another name for $B_6$.

■ *Physical Characteristics:* Knowing a vitamin when you eat one. . . . Some vitamins are carried in water and others in fat; some are destroyed by light and others by heat; some are green and others, orange. We tell all.

■ *Functions:* It's harder to ignore information when you know why it is important. . . . Each vitamin plays an important role in maintaining the health and well-being of both you and your baby. Knowing that folacin is necessary for cells to divide will help you select spinach—we hope.

■ *Dangers:* Too much or too little of a good thing . . . Not that we want to scare you, but you should know what current research shows about deficiencies and overdoses. Too much of some common vitamins can be *toxic*; that is, can cause permanent damage to you or your baby. Too little can cause a deficiency.

■ *Requirement During Pregnancy:* Then what *do* you need? There are the RDAs—but some people may need more. Do you?

■ *Food Sources:* Shopping for vitamins . . . The food sources lists will help you choose foods that you enjoy and encourage you to try some new ones. There may be some surprises.

■ *Getting the Maximum:* Vitamins are fragile! Even if you do not understand the technicalities, these tips will help you store, prepare, cook, and use vitamins so you get the most from them.

### Fat-Soluble Vitamins: A, D, E, and K

The *fat-soluble vitamins* are found mostly in fat or oil-containing foods. Some of the vitamins are used immediately; others are stored in fat "depots" in body tissue and in the liver. Because of these reserves, you do not need fat-soluble vitamins in your diet every day, though a consistently well-balanced diet will prevent the stores from becoming depleted. If excessive amounts of fat-soluble vitamins are consumed (especially A and D), the reserves become overly concentrated, and can be a threat to health.[50]

If you eat a reasonable diet, you will probably get adequate fat-soluble vitamins—unless you regularly use mineral oil or some other laxative. *Mineral oil* is not absorbed by the body, and will bind with fat-soluble vitamins, blocking their utilization and causing them to be excreted. Because fat-soluble vitamins are absorbed with fat, anything that interferes with the digestion of fat will decrease vitamin absorption.

There is a problem with measuring fat-soluble vitamins. We will explain it, for those who like mind-stretchers. For those who do not care about technicalities, the food sources of fat-soluble vitamins are clearly indicated in the following charts. Choose from these foods, and do not worry about the numbers!

Until recently, the term international units ("IU") was used in the United States to quantify fat-soluble vitamins. In 1980, the RDAs for fat-soluble vitamins were changed to correspond to what was used in most other countries.

Vitamins A and E are now measured in *retinol* and *tocopherol equivalents*, because these vitamins appear in several forms that are not all of equal strength. For example, the vitamin A in animal foods, called *retinol*, is six times more potent than *carotene*, the form of vitamin A in plant foods. Therefore, the measure of the vitamin is expressed as the amount equal to the vitamin A in one unit of retinol, an RE (retinol equivalent). Vitamins D and K now are expressed in *micrograms*. One microgram is equal to about forty of the former IUs.

## Water-Soluble Vitamins: C and B Vitamins

The *water-soluble vitamins* are quickly absorbed into the bloodstream and move through the body easily. Unlike the fat-soluble ones, they are not stored. Because what is not used in a relatively short time is generally excreted by the kidneys, concentrations in the blood do not build up. Nevertheless, the notion that very large amounts of water-soluble vitamins are safe is now being questioned, and excessive amounts are not recommended during pregnancy.

Excessive amounts of vitamin C, for example, can create problems because vitamin C can get trapped on the fetal side of the placenta and build up to high levels. The fetus can develop a dependency on a high concentration of the vitamin, which will result in discomfort at birth when the newborn must withdraw to levels found in breast milk or formula.[50]

Many American women have low levels of the B vitamins when they enter pregnancy. This is especially true of those who have been taking "the Pill." "The Pill" inhibits absorption of several of the B vitamins, a condition that can continue into pregnancy.

If you are pregnant, you need increased amounts of all the B vitamins. Several deserve special mention. The need for *folacin* (also called *folic acid* and *folate*) *doubles*, and there is research indicating unusually high demands for $B_6$ (*pyridoxine*) during pregnancy.[129] Vegetarians need to pay special attention to meeting $B_{12}$ needs.

The B vitamins work together as a team. Too much or too little of one or more can create an imbalance that reduces effectiveness. *Do not take large quantities of B-vitamin supplements during pregnancy without medical supervision.* Eat foods containing these vitamins, and consult your doctor about supplements—especially of folacin and $B_6$—to meet your individual needs.

# VITAMIN A

*Other Names*

Anti-infective
vitamin

Animal form:
Retinol

Vegetable form:
Carotene

*Physical
Characteristics*

Fat soluble

Fairly stable but
can be destroyed
by high tempera-
tures, air, sunlight,
drying

Carotene is an
orange pigment

*Functions*

Maintains epithelial
tissue (internal and
external "skin")—
there is over ¼ acre
in the adult.

Contributes to
development of
epithelial tissue
in fetus:
* Cornea (outside
covering of the eye)
* Linings of mouth,
sinuses, lungs,
digestive and
urinary tracts

Increases resistance
to infection

Promotes bone and
tooth development

Necessary for vision
in dim light

Related to hormone
production

*Dangers from
Too Much/Too Little*

Individual reactions to high
intakes. Pregnant women are
more sensitive to high levels
of vitamin A than non-
pregnant women.[46]

High levels can accumulate
to toxic levels in fetal bloodstream. Excesses have been
known to cause birth de-
fects.[50]

The symptoms of excessive
vitamin A intake are headache, nausea, diarrhea,
blurred vision, joint pain, loss
of appetite, stunted growth,
rashes, enlargement of liver,
and spleen.

Large amounts of retinol can
be toxic to mother. Huge
amounts of vitamin A from
carotene in vegetables cannot cause toxicity in any
amount.[147] Excesses will
cause skin to discolor.

Deficiency symptoms: poor
growth, infections, and eye
changes, which can cause
night blindness, eye disease,
and blindness.

# VITAMIN A *(cont.)*

*Requirement
During Pregnancy*

RDA = 1000 Retinol
Equivalents (RE).
Each RE is equal to
1 microgram of
retinol or 6 micro-
grams of carotene.
Carotene is ab-
sorbed less effec-
tively than retinol,
and must be con-
verted to active
retinol in the body
to be used.

*Food Sources*

Liver (because that's
where vitamin A is
stored in animals)

Fish-liver oils

*Color* is the key in
choosing foods rich
in vitamin A—bright
red, yellow, green,
and orange foods:
* Tomatoes
* Dark-green leafy
vegetables such as
spinach, broccoli,
greens (not iceberg
lettuce or celery)
* Deep-yellow or
orange vegetables
and fruits such as
carrots, squash,
apricots, pumpkins,
cantaloupe, sweet
potato, papaya

Milk

Cheese

Fortified margarine

Butter

*Getting the Maximum*

Vitamin A is relatively stable,
but can be destroyed when
exposed to heat and air. For
instance, vitamin A is greatly
diminished in oil after it has
been used for frying.

Vitamin A is contained in fat.
When fat is removed from
lowfat or skim milk, the vitamin A is also removed. If you
choose nonfat milk, be sure it
is fortified with vitamin A.

Vitamin A is well retained in
canned fruits and vegetables.
Tomato juice shows no loss of
this nutrient when canned.

Leaf lettuce and romaine contain more vitamin A than
their pale iceberg cousin.

Vitamin A is destroyed if rancidity occurs. Store oil and fat
in a cool, dark place. Do not
let butter or margarine stand
at room temperature for long
periods of time.

Mineral oil interferes with
absorption of vitamin A. (18)
Do not use mineral oil as a
laxative. Do not use low-
calorie salad dressings containing mineral oil.

# VITAMIN D

## Other Names

Calciferol

Several forms:
* Ergocalciferol ($D_2$)
* Cholecalciferol ($D_3$)
* Irradiated
  ergosterol
  (Irradiated means
  that the vitamin D
  was activated by
  exposure to light.
  Don't be concerned
  about radiation.)
* 7-dehydro-
  cholesterol
* Viosterol

## Physical Characteristics

Fat soluble

Generally stable

## Functions

Increases absorption and use of calcium and phosphorus, important for bone and tooth development of baby and maintenance of mother

Necessary for maintenance of normal levels of calcium and phosphorus in blood

## Danger from Too Much/Too Little

Women who have little exposure to sunlight, who live in areas of fog, or smog, or who have dark skin may have increased need.

Women who have had multiple pregnancies in a short period of time or who have breastfed for long periods just prior to this pregnancy may have depleted vitamin D stores.

Low levels of vitamin D may predispose a woman to tooth decay or soft bones that affect posture and cause lower back pain. Severe deficiency is rickets, characterized by bone deformities.

Maternal deficiency has been associated with seizures and rickets of newborns.[69]

Overdoses can occur with as little as four to five times daily need. Toxicity symptoms: calcium deposits in soft tissues, headache, diarrhea, nausea.

Excessive vitamin D can be toxic to the fetus and cause abnormal physical and mental development.[18]

*Requirement*
*During Pregnancy*

RDA:
* Under 18 years: 15 micrograms/
  day = 600 IU
* Ages 19–22: 12.5 micrograms/
  day = 500 IU
* Ages 23+: 10 micrograms/
  day = 400 IU

Additional vitamin D is required during pregnancy to prepare reserves for lactation and to form strong bones in the developing fetus.

If you drink enough vitamin D–fortified milk to meet your calcium need, the vitamin D will be provided as a bonus.

*Food*
*Sources*

There are only a few food sources of vitamin D:

Fortified milk
  (Approximately 98% of milk sold in the United States is fortified with vitamin D.)

Fortified margarine

Liver

Egg yolk

Fish-liver oils, such as tuna, cod, salmon

*Getting the*
*Maximum*

Vitamin D is formed in the skin when it is exposed to light. Sit in the sun!

Drink fortified milk.

# VITAMIN E

## Other Names

Tocopherol forms:
* Alpha-tocopherol
* Beta-tocopherol
* Delta-tocopherol
* Gamma-tocopherol

## Physical Characteristics

Fat soluble

Stable in heat, but not in air, freezing, or sunlight

## Functions

Antioxidant—protects vitamins A and C and polyunsaturated fats in the body from destruction by oxygen

Helps form normal blood cells, muscle cells, and other tissues

Appears to have effect on strength of membrane around red blood cells

There have been many claims for vitamin E. It is known as the antisterility vitamin, but it effects only rat fertility, not humans'! The relationship of vitamin E to a variety of other reproductive problems has not been documented for humans. [18]

Effectiveness in preventing permanent stretch marks has not been scientifically established

## Dangers from Too Much/ Too Little

Deficiency has not been seen in adults except when unable to absorb fats.

Toxicity not documented in humans. [46]

Little vitamin E crosses the placenta until late in pregnancy, so premature infants have a low supply.

- - - - - - - - - - - - - - - - - - - - - - - - - - - - - -

## Requirement During Pregnancy

RDA = 10 micrograms/ day, based on alpha-tocopherol equivalents.

Your body has great reserves of vitamin E in fatty tissues— supplements are not necessary.

## Food Sources

Vegetable oils

Whole grains (especially wheat germ)

Leafy vegetables

Mayonnaise

Seeds and nuts

Brown rice

Margarine

## Getting the Maximum

Vitamin E is destroyed in rancid oils. Store oils and fats and whole grains in cool, dark place such as refrigerator to prevent rancidity.

Needs increase as polyunsaturated fat sources increase, but these same sources supply the vitamin.

# VITAMIN K

| Other Names | Functions | Danger from Too Much/Too Little |
|---|---|---|
| Phylloquinone | Aids in blood clotting | Deficiency of vitamin K is unlikely except in newborn infants who cannot synthesize it. |
| Menaquinones | | |
| Menadione (a synthetic vitamin K) | | May be used by doctor during last few weeks of pregnancy or during labor to prevent hemorrhaging, but levels should be carefully controlled to prevent adverse reactions. |
| Former name: Antihemorrhagic vitamin | | |
| *Physical Characteristics* | | |
| Fat soluble | | |
| Heat stable | | Pregnant women and infants are prone to vitamin K toxicity.[46] Excesses can cause birth defects if taken in toxic dosage.[21] |
| Destroyed by light, strong acids | | |
| The synthetic form is water soluble | | |

| Requirement During Pregnancy | Food Sources | Getting the Maximum |
|---|---|---|
| Amount needed has been estimated to be 70–140 micrograms/day for an adult, but there is no daily recommendation because vitamin K is readily available in commonly eaten foods and is produced in the body by intestinal bacteria. | Dark-green leafy vegetables (best sources) | Store foods in a dark place, such as a refrigerator. |
| | Cabbage, broccoli | Stable; no losses in cooking. |
| | Liver | About half of the vitamin K you get is produced by bacteria normally present in the intestine, therefore antibiotics reduce synthesis. |
| Mothers who are being treated with antibiotics may need supplements, because antibiotics reduce ability of gastrointestinal tract to produce vitamin K. | Egg yolk | |
| | Cauliflower | |
| Chronic diarrhea or poor absorption may increase need. | Tomatoes | Aspirin interferes with utilization of vitamin K.[136] |
| Vitamin K may be given to newborns to prevent bleeding. | | |

# VITAMIN C

*Other Name*

Ascorbic acid

*Physical Characteristics*

Water soluble

The least stable of vitamins; destroyed by air when in liquids

Destruction accelerated by light and by exposure to some metals

*Functions*

Necessary for normal functioning of all cells

Vitamin C is essential for development of bones, teeth, blood vessels. It is necessary for the formation of collagen, which holds skin and bones together—sometimes called "cell cement."

Vitamin C increases absorption of iron from food —important during pregnancy because iron is needed for the increased blood volume.

Converts inactive form of folic acid to active form needed for blood cells.

There is controversy over the role of vitamin C in preventing illness, such as colds, but there is agreement on its importance in the healing process.

Added to foods vitamin C is a preservative.

*Dangers from Too Much/Too Little*

Megadoses of vitamin C during pregnancy can condition the child to greater need *after* birth. A newborn will experience temporary (but painful) deficiency when given only breast milk or formula until the baby adjusts to more normal levels.[50] This is called "rebound scurvy."

Symptoms of excessive intake are diarrhea, rashes, frequent urination; high intake can cause kidney stones and gout in some individuals.

Symptoms of mild deficiency are bleeding gums, easy bruising, slow healing, weakness, aches, and bone pain. Severe deficiency is called scurvy.

Low maternal intakes associated with increased death rates of newborns.[18]

# VITAMIN C *(cont.)*

*Requirement During Pregnancy*

RDAs are increased by 20 milligrams, to 80 milligrams/day, during pregnancy to meet the demands for fetal growth and maternal tissues.

Vitamin C must be provided each day.

Women who smoke cigarettes have an increased need for vitamin C. This need can be met by drinking one 8-ounce glass of orange juice (100 milligrams of vitamin C) each day.

*Food Sources*

Almost exclusively from fruits and vegetables:

Citrus fruits, juices

Acerola cherry

Green peppers

Berries

Tomatoes and tomato juice

Brussels sprouts

Melons, cantaloupe

Mangos, papaya

Broccoli

Cabbage

Pineapple

Cauliflower

Spinach, kale

Turnips

Potatoes

Mustard, collard greens

*Getting the Maximum*

Vitamin C is the most perishable of all vitamins.

Store foods in cool, dark place.

Do not cut or peel fruits and vegetables until ready to serve; bake potatoes whole.

Store juices in covered containers.

Cook vegetables quickly or steam them.

Dried fruits have practically no vitamin C.

Excretion increases with some medications (steroids, antibiotics, salicylates such as aspirin).

Extreme stress places demands on vitamin C.

# THE B VITAMINS: Thiamin

**Other Names**

B₁

Former names
* Vitamin F
* Antiberiberi factor

*Physical
Characteristics*

Water soluble

Stable in heat when
dry or in acid;
destroyed in alka-
line solutions

Destroyed when
exposed to air

Nutlike or yeasty in
odor and flavor

*Functions*

Promotes change
of carbohydrates
into energy

Aids in digestion

Related to normal
appetite

Essential for func-
tioning of nerv-
vous system

Maintains muscle
tone for heart
function

Role in metab-
olism of fat

*Danger from
Too Much/Too Little*

Carbohydrate is essential for
fetal brain development, and
thiamin is essential for carbohydrate to be used for this task.
Thiamin must be supplied or
brain development will be im-
paired.

Thiamin is called the "morale
vitamin" because deficiency
can cause depression or irritability. Other symptoms of deficiency are loss of appetite,
fatigue, constipation, backache,
insomnia, cramps. All of the
above "symptoms" are common
during pregnancy, and may not
necessarily be caused by a thiamin deficiency.

Classic deficiency is beriberi,
which is characterized by
nausea, irritability, poor appetite, confusion, fatigue,
muscle aches, and damage to
the nervous system leading to
paralysis.

Deficiencies are most commonly
associated with high alcohol
consumption.

| *Requirement During Pregnancy* | *Food Sources* | *Getting the Maximum* |
|---|---|---|
| RDA = 1.5 milligrams/day | Lean pork (best source) | Refined carbohydrates such as sugar or alcohol contain no thiamin, but require thiamin for metabolism—another reason to limit consumption of these foods. |
| Thiamin needs depend on caloric intake because thiamin is needed to utilize the carbohydrate that provides calories. | Liver<br><br>Lean meat<br><br>Brewer's yeast<br><br>Fish | Most excellent sources of thiamin are in meat. Vegetarians who eat plenty of whole grains and enriched breads and cereals can get adequate thiamin. |
| If you were underweight or undernourished before pregnancy, and have been encouraged to increase your calorie intake above normal recommendations for your age during pregnancy, you will also need more thiamin. | Legumes, peas, soybeans<br><br>Enriched or whole-grain breads, cereals (Enriched grains have restored levels of the thiamin lost in processing.) | Do not wash rice before cooking.<br><br>Cook vegetables in as little water as possible.<br><br>Do not add baking soda to water when cooking beans, greens, or any vegetable—it destroys the vitamin.<br><br>Overcooking beef destroys thiamin. |
| Some studies indicate thiamin may relieve nausea in pregnancy.[18] | Nuts, especially Brazil nuts<br><br>Asparagus<br><br>Wheat germ | Use of antacids for control of nausea reduces utilization of thiamin.<br><br>Some diuretic medications increase urinary loss of thiamin. |

# THE B VITAMINS: Riboflavin

*Other Names*

B₂

Former name:
Vitamin G

*Physical
Characteristics*

Water soluble

Yellow-green
fluorescent color

Relatively heat
stable. Stable in
oxygen; unstable
in light and alkali.

*Functions*

Essential for release of
energy from carbohydrates,
fat, and protein

Necessary for growth

Promotes good vision and
healthy skin

Necessary for conversion of
tryptophan to niacin

*Dangers from
Too Much/Too Little*

Animal studies have
shown that lack of ribo-
flavin in thirteenth
and fourteenth embry-
onic days can lead to
bone and organ mal-
formations.[18]

Lack of riboflavin was
once thought to cause
prematurity, but recent
studies show no corre-
lation.[50]

Symptoms of deficiency
include cracked and
sore mouth, watery
bloodshot eyes, swol-
len tongue.

No known danger from
excesses.

| Requirement During Pregnancy | Food Sources | Getting the Maximum |
|---|---|---|
| RDA = 1.5 to 1.6 milligrams/day | About half of riboflavin comes from dairy products; 25 percent from meat. | Store milk away from light in an opaque container. Milk exposed to sunlight for several hours can lose 50–70 percent of the riboflavin. |
| Strict vegetarians may have difficulty meeting needs. | Milk | |
| | Yogurt | |
| | Cheese | Do not add baking soda to water when cooking greens or beans. |
| | Organ meats, liver (including chicken livers) | |
| | Lean meat | Certain diuretics and antibiotics can increase urinary excretion of the vitamin. |
| | Leafy green vegetables (especially spinach, asparagus) | |
| | Whole grains, barley | |
| | Enriched breads, cereals (Enriched grains have added riboflavin, lost in processing from whole grain.) | |
| | Brewer's yeast | |
| | Dried peas and beans | |
| | Peanuts | |

# THE B VITAMINS: Niacin

**Other Names**

$B_3$

Nicotinic acid*

Nicotinamide*

Niacinamide

*Not the same as
nicotine in cigarettes.

*Physical Characteristics*

Water soluble

One of the most stable of
the B vitamins

Destroyed by light

**Functions**

Needed for conversion of glucose to energy

Present in all body tissues, and therefore very important to total growth and development of fetus

Promotes healthy skin, nerves, digestive tract

**Dangers from Too Much/Too Little**

Niacin deficiency is uncommon in people who eat complete and adequate protein, especially from meat and milk.

Effects of niacin deficiency in pregnant women have not been thoroughly investigated.

Alcoholics may suffer niacin deficiency.

Diets high in corn and cornmeal can contribute to deficiency.

Deficiency (pellegra) marked by irritability, loss of appetite, swollen tongue, insomnia, skin rash, headache, digestive disorders.

# THE B VITAMINS: Niacin *(cont.)*

*Requirement
During Pregnancy*

Ages 16–22: 16 Niacin
  Equivalents/day
Ages 23+: 15 Niacin
  Equivalents/day

You may see the term
"Niacin Equivalents" (NEs)
used to describe amounts
of niacin. Niacin can be
converted from trypto-
phan, an amino acid that
is present in all complete
proteins. So the Niacin
Equivalents equal the
amount of niacin itself plus
the amount formed from
the tryptophan.

*Food Sources*

Complete pro-
teins: liver, lean
meat, poultry,
fish, eggs

Brewer's yeast

Whole and en-
riched grains,
especially bran

Legumes, pinto
beans, peas,
peanuts, peanut
butter

*Getting the Maximum*

Losses in cooking are due
largely to the fact that the
vitamin is water soluble.
Use as little water as possible in cooking.

Do not completely thaw
frozen fish before cooking.
Niacin is lost if liquid from
fish is discarded.

# THE B VITAMINS: Vitamin B$_6$

| Other Names | Functions | Dangers from Too Much/Too Little |
|---|---|---|
| Pyridoxine | Involved in protein and fat utilization | Women who have taken "the Pill" until just prior to pregnancy may have difficulty absorbing vitamin B$_6$, increasing their need. |
| Pyridoxal | | |
| Pyridoxamine | Supports energy-producing system in the body | |
| *Physical Characteristics* | | Symptoms of deficiency are anemia, nervousness, dry mouth, weakness, nausea, tingling sensation in fingers and toes. All of the above "symptoms" are common during pregnancy, and are not necessarily caused by a B$_6$ deficiency. |
| Water soluble | Especially important for development of fetal brain and nerve tissue | |
| Generally stable; can be destroyed by light and heat | | |
| | Necessary for conversion of tryptophan to niacin. | |
| | Affects hormones, related to stress | Large supplements may condition the fetus to high intakes and cause withdrawal problems after birth.[18] |
| | Necessary for absorption of some amino acids | |
| | Associated with immunity to disease | |

# THE B VITAMINS: Vitamin B$_6$ *(cont.)*

*Requirement*
*During Pregnancy*

RDA = 2.6 milligrams/day
Need is related to protein
intake.

Some B$_6$ can be made in
the digestive tract.

Needs are increased dur-
ing pregnancy because
the fetus has high demand
for B$_6$ (about five times that
of the mother).

There is mixed evidence
about the value of supplements. The National Re-
search Council does not
believe they are justified;[6]
others say supplements
may be necessary to meet
fetal demands.[100]

Talk with your doctor
about the adequacy of
your diet to meet your
individual needs.

B$_6$ may be prescribed by
doctor for relief of nausea
or vomiting during preg-
nancy (50 mg/day). There
has been limited success
with this treatment.[107]

*Food Sources*

Wheat germ

Meat, especially
liver, kidney

Whole-grain
cereals, bread

Bananas

Beans, peas,
soybeans

Nuts and seeds

Corn

Poultry

Fish

Vegetables, es-
pecially green
leafy vegetables

Avocado

Cabbage

Bran

Yams

*Getting the Maximum*

Eat whole-grain cereals
and breads. Up to 90 per-
cent of B$_6$ is destroyed by
processing, and is not replaced by enrichment.[50]

B$_6$ in vegetable sources is
more resistant to losses
than animal sources of
the vitamin; include fresh
vegetables in your daily
diet.

Some medications, such
as those used to treat
tuberculosis, interfere with
B$_6$.

# THE B VITAMINS: Vitamin B₁₂

*Other Names*

Cobalamin

Extrinsic factor

*Physical Characteristics*

Water soluble

Destroyed by heat and light

Red-colored

Only vitamin known to contain the mineral cobalt

*Functions*

Necessary for formation of proteins

Important for red-blood-cell formation—especially important for development and function of brain and nerve cells

Essential for cell division and growth.

*Dangers from Too Much/Too Little*

Chronic deficiency (pernicious anemia) is dangerous because it can cause irreparable damage to the nervous system. This is rare except among strict vegetarians, alcoholics, and some receiving certain medications.

Deficiencies develop very slowly and are hard to detect.

$B_{12}$ needs secretions from the stomach wall to be absorbed. If there is a malfunction of this mechanism, a deficiency may occur. This is more likely to be the cause of a deficiency than a lack of $B_{12}$ in the diet. Your doctor is responsible for detecting this problem.

Low levels of $B_{12}$ are associated with premature birth; especially true of babies born to women who smoke.[18]

Long-term antibiotic treatments can lead to $B_{12}$ deficiency.

No known toxicity.

*Requirement
During Pregnancy*

RDA = 4 micrograms/day. This allows for a margin of safety for individual absorption variations.

Though most water-soluble vitamins are excreted in urine if excessive, $B_{12}$ is bound to a protein and stored in the body. The fetus can draw on these reserves.

$B_{12}$ supplements are recommended for vegetarians.

*Food Sources*

Found almost exclusively in animal foods:
* Liver
* Kidney
* Lean meats
* Fish
* Oysters, clams
* Cheese (especially cottage cheese)
* Egg yolk

Sauerkraut

Pineapple

Tofu (soybean curd)

*Getting the Maximum*

More $B_{12}$ is absorbed during pregnancy.

Pasteurization reduces amount of $B_{12}$ in milk. Boiling milk for long periods of time will reduce $B_{12}$.

Factors that decrease absorption of $B_{12}$:
* lack of secretions in stomach
* gastrointestinal problems

# THE B VITAMINS: Folacin

## Other Names

Folic acid

Folate

Pteroylglutamic
acid (PGA)

Former names:
* Vitamin M
* Citrovorum factor

## Physical Characteristics

Deteriorates at room
temperature and in
sunlight

Destroyed by high
heat

## Functions

Folacin is neces-
sary for cell divi-
sion—the basis of
growth of the
fetus.

Essential compo-
nent of blood cells
and enzymes

Folacin is impor-
tant in increasing
number of blood
cells.

Necessary for
utilization of
some amino
acids

## Dangers from Too Much/Too Little

Deficiency causes anemia in
the mother. Some studies suggest that deficiency correlates
with spontaneous abortion. Most
medical opinion is that deficiency is unlikely to cause complications other than maternal
anemia. [130]

Though there is little chance of
toxicity from large doses, large
amounts are not given because
it can "mask" detection of $B_{12}$
deficiency. For this reason the
Food and Drug Administration
has set limits on the amount of
folacin, per tablet, that can be
sold without a doctor's prescription.

Certain medications may interfere with folacin utilization.

Oral contraceptives and hormonal changes of pregnancy
produce decreased levels in
blood tests. How much is optimal
in pregnancy has not been
agreed upon by medical
authorities.

# THE B VITAMINS: Folacin *(cont.)*

*Requirement During Pregnancy*

RDA = 800 micrograms/day

The need in pregnancy doubles.

Prenatal vitamin supplements have more folacin than regular multivitamins.

Some folacin is synthesized by bacteria in the intestines.

Because optimal levels of intake are not well understood, oral supplements may be given.

*Food Sources*

Leafy green vegetables (spinach, greens, romaine lettuce)

Liver, kidney

Brewer's yeast

Legumes: garbanzos and kidney beans

Nuts

Mushrooms

Asparagus

Broccoli

Orange juice

Lemons

Strawberries

Potatoes

Eggs

Cantaloupe

Beets

Avocados

*Getting the Maximum*

Folacin is stable in orange juice because it is protected by vitamin C.

Eat fruits and vegetables raw for maximum benefit.

Folacin is lost whenever high temperature or large amounts of water are used in cooking.

Refrigerate fruits and vegetables to prevent loss of the vitamin.

Chronic alcoholics cannot absorb the common dietary forms of folacin. The synthetic form of the vitamin is better utilized.

More folacin is destroyed by microwave cooking than by other cooking methods.

# THE B VITAMINS: Pantothenic Acid

*Other Names*

None

*Physical Characteristics*

Water soluble

Readily destroyed in dry heat, but not in moist heat

Can be destroyed by alkali or acid

*Functions*

Essential for metabolism of carbohydrate and protein from foods into substances that can be used in the human body

Necessary to make hormones

Formation of pigment in hemoglobin (makes red blood red)

*Dangers from Too Much/Too Little*

Severe deficiencies are infrequent in humans except for those under extreme stress, but low intake can lower resistance to infection and increase irritability, cramps, fatigue, depression, and burning feeling in feet.

Pantothenic acid will *not* prevent hair from turning gray. That is a myth.

- - - - - - - - - - - - - - - - - - - - - - - - - - - - - -

*Requirement During Pregnancy*

No specific RDA has been established, but needs are estimated to be 4 to 7 milligrams/day

Supplements are not necessary because foods provide a ready source.

Some pantothenic acid is made in the digestive tract.

*Food Sources*

Pantothenic acid is found in all living matter.

Beef liver, kidney

Fish, salmon

Whole grains

Egg yolk

Most vegetables

Nuts

Poultry

*Getting the Maximum*

Canning destroys 20–35 percent of the vitamin in animal foods and up to 75 percent in vegetable foods. It is better to choose fresh or frozen vegetables.

Forty percent is lost in refining wheat—choose whole-grain cereals and breads.

# THE B VITAMINS: Biotin

### Other Names

Former names:
Vitamin H

Co-enzyme R

### Physical Characteristics

Water soluble

Stable in heat, acid

Readily destroyed by air and light

### Functions

Necessary for release of energy from other nutrients

Necessary for synthesis of some fats

### Dangers from Too Much/Too Little

Deficiency in man causes specific types of skin problems, loss of appetite, muscle pain, nausea.

No know risks from excesses.

- - - - - - - - - - - - - - - - - - - - - - - - - - - - - - - - - - -

### Requirement During Pregnancy

100 to 200 micrograms/day is estimated to be adequate.

Most diets contain 150 to 300 micrograms of biotin daily—enough to meet the needs of pregnancy.

Some biotin is made in the digestive tract.

### Food Sources

Biotin is present in most foods.

Egg yolk

Liver

Kidney

Cauliflower

Mushrooms

Dried peas and beans, soybeans

Nuts

### Getting the Maximum

Curiously, biotin is destroyed by raw egg whites, but it would take a diet of twenty-five to thirty raw egg whites a day (30 percent of your total diet) to cause any problem. Cooking egg whites renders them harmless.

Some biotin may be lost in cooking water—again, the less water you use in cooking, the better.

Some biotin is synthesized by bacteria in the intestine; taking antibiotics reduces this production.

## The Un-Vitamins

There are many substances that are not currently considered vitamins, but that have some vitaminlike characteristics. These are promoted by many magazines and salespeople as essential to health. They do not have unique biological functions in humans. Some of these pseudo-vitamins, including those listed below and others such as ubiquinone, lipoic acid, and bioflavonoids are produced by the body in adequate amounts or are merely part of other substances. Deficiencies are not known and supplementation is unnecessary.

*Para-Aminobenzoic Acid (PABA)* was formerly thought to be a vitamin for humans. Now we know that it is a part of folacin.

*Choline* is produced by both plants and animals, including humans. It is a component of many body compounds. Food sources include egg yolk, organ meat, wheat germ, and legumes. Typical diets provide plenty of choline.

*Inositol* is a component of fatlike substances in muscles. Deficiencies are unknown. It is widely available in grains, nuts, fruits, vegetables, yeast, and milk.

*Pangamic Acid* (also called Vitamin $B_{15}$) is described by Dr. Victor Herbert, a dynamic crusader against food fraud, and past president of the American Society for Clinical Nutrition, this way: "Pangamic acid is a loose term which most often describes a substance which is one part sodium (or calcium) gluconate, one part glycine (or dimethyl glycine), one part diisopropylamine dichloroacetate, and no part vitamin. It is deceptively and misleadingly trade-named 'vitamin $B_{15}$.' But it is nutritionally worthless. It has no vitamin properties, and no such vitamin exists."[87]

*Laetrile* (also called Vitamin $B_{17}$) has been promoted as a cancer preventative and cure. The anti-cancer effectiveness of laetrile has not been substantiated. It is a harmful substance containing cyanide, which destroys cells. It should *never* be taken by a pregnant woman.

# 6.
# Minerals:
# The Strong Supports

95

When you build a home, you want the supports to be strong and durable. The strength and durability of materials that support the human body are equally important. Minerals meet these specifications, serving as the support structure of your body and your baby's body. Minerals are not needed in large amounts, but when you understand the important role they play, you'll see that this is no place to "cut corners" when it comes to baby-building.

Most of the mineral "deposits" in humans are found in bones and teeth, which survive after the rest of the body is long gone. Sugar and spice are very nice and snips and snails and puppy dog tails make good nursery rhymes—but *minerals* are what healthy boys and girls are really made of!

Minerals are strong and durable, in part, because they are elements. An *element* consists of a single kind of atom, the basic building blocks of all matter. Not only can minerals not be broken into chemical parts, they cannot be destroyed.

Minerals used by the human body must be provided by the diet—they are not manufactured internally. During pregnancy, when you are helping to build a new body and maintaining your own, an adequate supply of minerals is essential.

*Minerals have two functions—building and regulating.* As builders, minerals help form the skeleton and all soft tissues, and they help form parts of vital body chemicals—such as iron in the hemoglobin of red blood cells and iodine in the thyroid hormone, thyroxine. As regulators, minerals can influence a wide variety of systems such as heartbeat, blood clotting, maintenance of the pressure of body fluids, nerve behavior, and transport of oxygen from lungs to tissues. A simplified explanation of how minerals build and regulate is fascinating.

Regulatory functions are frequently performed by minerals with electrical charges, called *ions*. Like magnets, some of these electrically charged minerals have minus charges; other ions have plus charges. The actions of these ions help regulate many body systems.

There are body fluids both inside and outside your body's

cells. The balance of plus- and minus-charged ions keeps the fluid outside the cells from putting too much pressure on them, and also maintains a fluid pressure inside the cells that is great enough to keep the cells from collapsing. This balance of fluids inside and outside the body cells helps make it physically possible for humans to live on land.

Some minerals are found in significant quantities in the body. These *macrominerals* are *calcium, phosphorus, sodium, chloride, potassium, magnesium,* and *sulfur.* Others, equally essential, though present in extremely small quantities, are called *microminerals* or, more commonly, *trace minerals* or *trace elements.* They are *iron, chromium, cobalt, copper, fluoride, iodine, vanadium, manganese, molybdenum, nickel, selenium, silicon, tin,* and *zinc.* Many other minerals occur in nature that are not needed by the human body. Some of these, such as lead, cadmium, and mercury, are harmful or fatal if consumed in large amounts.

## The Macrominerals

### Calcium and Phosphorus: Team Players

We tend to think of bones as unchanging structures. Most people don't realize that bones are constantly being broken down and rebuilt. Minerals are lost from bones when calcium and phosphorus are released to regulate nerve and muscle activity, including heartbeat, blood clotting, and cell membrane integrity.

During pregnancy, the minerals in your bones may also be used to build the baby's skeleton. The minerals for the baby *should* come from the food you eat. *If the minerals in your diet are inadequate, your bones may have to give up their minerals to help build your baby's bones and teeth.*

Mother Nature makes the most of what she has to work with:

* by increasing the efficiency of absorption. You absorb more calcium from a glass of milk when you are pregnant than when you are not pregnant;

* by increasing the release of calcium from bones, if it is needed;
* by encouraging the deposit of calcium to build your baby's bones.

---

Many women do not consume recommended amounts of calcium even before they become pregnant. During pregnancy, you must dramatically increase your calcium consumption to provide sufficient calcium to meet the baby's needs as well as your own. If you plan to breastfeed, you need to prepare for this, too. Almost all of the extra calcium needed during pregnancy is used by the baby. During the last trimester, 200 to 300 milligrams of calcium is deposited in the baby *each day*. If your diet isn't equal to the task, your bones will give up their calcium and phosphorus to help satisfy your baby's needs.

Some people will tell you that the extraordinary demand for calcium causes *tooth decay* because calcium is drawn from the mother's teeth. No studies have confirmed this, however. Calcium can be drawn from the mother's *bones*, but not her teeth. The slight increase in cavities during pregnancy that some people report may be due to a minor change in the composition of the saliva in the mouth. This potential problem can be dealt with by practicing good dental hygiene.

Calcium and phosphorus work as a team. They are absorbed and deposited in bones in combination with each other. Vitamin D increases the efficiency of this partnership. It is apparent that the *combination of nutrients in milk is the easiest and most efficient way to meet your calcium-phosphorus needs*.

Dr. Roy Pitkin, a prominent researcher in prenatal nutrition, in discussing calcium needs, recently stated: "Since it is virtually impossible to meet these requirements with natural foods other than dairy products, milk is considered by many to be practically essential for the pregnant woman. The allowance for pregnancy—1,200 mg—is precisely that contained in one quart of milk. Individuals who do not consume milk or milk products will require calcium supplementation."[128]

Drinking milk during pregnancy is not universally recommended. Our friend Betsy recounts her experience: "For my first pregnancy, I went to a doctor who told me I'd be a 'sorry sow' afterward if I didn't 'watch my weight,' and definitely not to drink milk because 'that's what makes you fat.' I gained 41 pounds and had a beautiful 7½-pound daughter, who at four years old had four cavities to be filled and is very small for her age. The second pregnancy was with a different group of doctors who were not at all concerned with Mother's weight and who encouraged drinking a quart of milk a day. Fifty pounds later, I delivered a beautiful 9-pound daughter. We'll see how many fillings she needs at four.... Meanwhile, two months later I've lost 30 pounds and look like Miss Piggy."

Mary, with experience in nutrition counseling, comments: "Milk—or any other food, for that matter—does not cause weight gain. Calories cause weight gain. If you increase the amount of milk you drink when you are pregnant, you are also increasing the number of calories you consume.

"Evaluate your total diet to see if your intake of calories exceeds your needs. If so, eliminate other less nutritious sources of calories before you decide to give up milk. If weight gain is a problem, choose skim milk.

"Betsy's weight gain during both pregnancies was higher than usual—with milk and without. She had no pregnancy complications and easy labors and deliveries. Betsy has had problems controlling her weight even when she has not been pregnant. The reality is, if you gain more than 30 or 35 pounds, it will probably take some time and exercise to get it off!"

Milk and dairy products provide about 85 percent of the calcium consumed in the United States. Although drinking milk is not essential to an adequate diet during pregnancy, it certainly simplifies meeting a variety of nutrient needs, not only for calcium and phosphorus, but also for protein, riboflavin, vitamin $B_{12}$, vitamin D, and many other nutrients.

Calcium is aided in both absorption and utilization by vitamin D in fortified milk and milk products. Vitamin D helps the calcium get out of your digestive tract and into your bloodstream. A severe calcium deficiency can be caused by either a deficiency of vitamin D or a deficiency of dietary calcium. Huge amounts of vitamin D can lead to excessive absorption of calcium, which can cause irregular fetal bone formation.

Calcium absorption is also improved by *lactose* or *milk sugar*, a carbohydrate found in milk. Some women, unable to digest lactose, get diarrhea if they drink milk. Fermented dairy products, such as buttermilk, yogurt and natural cheeses, contain less lactose, and may be used instead of milk to provide the nutrients we've been talking about, but if cheese is chosen, additional fluids are needed to replace the liquid in milk.

Agnes Higgins, director of the Montreal Diet Dispensary, tells her patients to drink milk at regular intervals because the baby is growing at a rate even more rapid than that after birth, and needs to be "fed" frequently. Milk, she says, is the perfect food for the baby, both before and after birth. Even women who have never been able to drink milk find they can do so under Mrs. Higgins' urging to "Feed the baby! Just because you can't hear him crying doesn't mean he isn't hungry."[172] Mrs. Higgins may be stretching the physical facts a bit to make her point, but her enthusiasm about drinking milk during pregnancy is justifiable. A milk-fed fetus is more likely to be what Mrs. Higgins calls "a Blue Ribbon Baby" than one that depends on less reliable sources of nutrients.

A total of 1,200 milligrams of calcium a day is generally recommended for the healthy pregnant adult woman (more is needed by pregnant teens). One cup of milk contains 300 milligrams. *If you drink a quart of milk a day when you are pregnant, you are giving your baby its calcium.* It does not matter whether you eat yogurt or drink whole milk, skim milk, reconstituted dry milk, or buttermilk—the calcium is still there. Butter and cream, however, are *not* good sources of calcium. You don't have to drink your milk from a glass, either. You can put it into pancakes, soups, casseroles, or puddings.

Some people like to add a bit of vanilla and a dash of cinnamon for a different taste. The addition of chocolate reduces the amount of calcium absorption somewhat, but if the only way you can stand to drink milk is to flavor it, that's better than not drinking it at all.

For a variety of reasons, including intolerance to milk, some women must rely on alternative calcium sources. If you are unable to drink milk for any reason, be sure to tell your doctor. Probably a calcium supplement will be prescribed along with a recommendation to increase the consumption of non-milk calcium sources.

The following chart identifies sources of calcium that arε equivalent to one cup of milk. If canned fish is eaten to meet calcium needs, it must be eaten with its soft edible bones; canned tuna or whole fish without bones is low in calcium.

| CALCIUM SOURCES [34] | |
|---|---|
| Foods | Amounts equivalent to 1 cup milk |
| Almonds | 1 cup |
| Broccoli, cooked | 2½ cups, 3 stalks |
| Cheddar cheese | 1½ oz. |
| Collard greens, cooked, chopped | 1 cup |
| Cottage cheese, creamed | 1½ cups |
| Kale, cooked | 1¾ cups |
| Mackerel, canned | 4 oz. |
| Mozzarella cheese | 4 oz. |
| Sardines, canned | 7 medium |
| Tofu, soybean curd | 8 oz. |
| Turnip greens, cooked | 1 cup |
| Yogurt | 1 cup |

## Phosphorus

Phosphorus is the vice-presidential mineral. Many people have never even heard of it, while others would be hard-pressed to describe it.

And yet, there is no substitute for phosphorus. Without it, bones and teeth would not grow strong and rigid, calcium absorption would be diminished, new cell growth could not take place, B vitamins could not work properly, the body could not produce energy from glucose, blood composition and balance would change, and fat could not be transported.

The recommendation for phosphorus intake during pregnancy is the same as for calcium—1,200 milligrams a day. Each is absorbed better if accompanied by the other and by vitamin D. All three of these nutrients are plentiful in milk and dairy products.

The American diet includes a great deal of phosphorus in foods that do not contain calcium or vitamin D—and this may cause problems if calcium recommendations are not met. Forms of phosphorus (usually phosphates) are abundant in snack foods, soft drinks, processed meats; because phosphorus is found in muscles, it is also in lean red meat. Most women can tolerate wide variations in the relationship of phosphorus to calcium, if there is adequate vitamin D. But during pregnancy, you want to improve the body's use of calcium, which can be hampered by the consumption of too much phosphorus and not enough calcium.

Sudden leg cramps are a common problem late in pregnancy. This may be due to an imbalance of calcium and phosphorus. Prevention and relief of leg cramps is discussed in Chapter 9.

### The Ins and Outs of Sodium, Potassium, and Chloride

That business about pregnant women craving pickles may not be so crazy, after all. Pickles contain a lot of salt—and salt is a vital nutrient during pregnancy. When the blood levels of salt fall, humans and some other animals, too, have a "taste for salt."

During pregnancy, changes take place that necessitate an increased need for salt. Since increasing salt intake counters advice being given the general public to reduce the amount of salt consumed, and since you may have been told to restrict salt during pregnancy to prevent weight gain or toxemia, an understanding of the increased salt requirement of pregnancy deserves special attention.

*Salt* is a combination of the minerals *sodium* and *chloride*. Because sodium is a plus ion and chloride is a minus ion, they are attracted to each other as a dry substance and form a very durable bond—until they are put into a liquid, at which time they separate and return to their ion forms. In the body, salt enters the bloodstream, a water-based liquid, and from there on, sodium and chloride go about performing their separate but integrated jobs. Along with the mineral potassium, they help regulate fluids in our cells and throughout our bodies.

One principle behind fluid balance control is that water "follows" sodium. If you have ever sprinkled salt on cucumbers, you have seen this mechanism work. After a few minutes, the salt draws liquid out of the cucumbers. Sodium, in the fluid outside the body cells, draws water out of the cells in a similar way. If it were not for potassium and chloride inside the cells, you would be left with cells that are limp as salted cucumbers!

Some people seem very sensitive to salt. If they consume excessive amounts of salt, the cell floodgates cannot hold back the water, and the water is drawn into the bloodstream. As the volume of fluid in the blood increases, blood pressure increases. This condition is known as *hypertension* or *high blood pressure*.

During pregnancy, however, the blood volume normally increases about 33 percent. This is necessary to provide adequate flow of blood to your baby. As the blood volume expands, the amount of water held in reserve in cells also expands. Sometimes, the cells get so full that they swell. This swelling is called *edema*. Some degree of edema is normal during pregnancy (see Chapter 9).

*The normal edema of pregnancy should not be treated by restricting salt, or with diuretics (water pills), which are designed to eliminate water from the body.* You need the added fluid during pregnancy, and the added fluid requires increased amounts of minerals such as sodium, potassium, and chloride.

If edema becomes excessive, there is usually a medical reason. It is a symptom of several serious problems and you should be examined by your doctor.

Until recently, there has been little evidence to support a specific recommendation for a pregnant woman's daily salt intake. *Current medical opinion holds that pregnant women should not limit salt and should salt food "to taste."* The amount of sodium that you need can be obtained from a varied diet without any effort to restrict or increase salt intake.[130]

No RDAs for sodium or chloride have been established but safe and adequate levels of intake have been determined. Both of these nutrients are easy to get because they are widely available in many foods. Most of us are aware of the high levels of salt in some processed foods; in addition, some sodium occurs naturally in foods. The salt consumption of many Americans is more than is desirable. Individuals with a tendency toward hypertension may need to restrict foods high in salt. If you have hypertension, your doctor will monitor your pregnancy with particular care. But, in general, pregnancy is not a time to restrict salt.

Like sodium and chloride, *potassium* helps regulate fluid balance and fluid volume in cells. It also is vital to the action of the heart. Unless you sweat profusely, day after day, or you are taking medication that causes potassium loss, your food supply should be adequate to meet your need for potassium during pregnancy. Potassium deficiencies are virtually unknown in this country, except as a result of severe vomiting, protein-malnutrition, or when diuretics have been excessively used. The amount of potassium usually consumed is readily available in the diet, and is sufficient to meet the needs of pregnancy.

Megadoses of potassium supplements can cause imbalances leading to muscular paralysis and abnormal heartbeat rhythm. There is a reported case of a two-month-old infant who died from being given liquid potassium supplements to treat colic—a treatment suggested by the late Adelle Davis.[8] This case is mentioned to illustrate the potential dangers of supplementing your own or your child's diet.

### POTASSIUM SOURCES

| | |
|---|---|
| Apricots, dried | Milk |
| Avocados | Most fruits |
| Bananas | Most vegetables |
| Cantaloupe | Oranges and juice |
| Chicken | Peanut butter |
| Meat | Potatoes |

## The Last (Sulfur) and the Least (Magnesium) of the Macronutrients

There is *sulfur* in every cell in the body. It is a structural component of the proteins in hair, skin, and nails. (If you have ever smelled burning hair, the strange odor is sulfur dioxide.) Sulfur is contained in several vitamins (thiamin and biotin) and in methionine, an amino acid.

If your diet contains adequate protein, you will receive sufficient sulfur to meet the needs of pregnancy. Eggs, meat, milk, cheese, nuts, and legumes all have lots of sulfur.

*Magnesium* almost doesn't make it as a macromineral because it is present in such small quantities. Deficiencies, while uncommon, are recognized by a lack of neuromuscular control. Magnesium is stored in bones, and is released when needed to assist in the release of energy, to help utilize protein, and to allow muscles to contract.

The RDA for magnesium of 300 milligrams a day for women is sufficient to meet the needs of pregnancy. Magnesium is an essential part of chlorophyll, the green pigment in plants. Green leafy vegetables containing chlorophyll are excellent sources of magnesium. Other magnesium-containing foods are meat, bran, wheat germ, cocoa, nuts, soybeans, and whole grains.

If your diet is adequate in calories and protein, you are getting enough magnesium. If, on the other hand, you have suffered from prolonged diarrhea or vomiting, or have made extensive use of diuretics, you may need to make a special effort to include magnesium-rich foods in your diet.

## The Trace Minerals

All living matter, including the human body, contains tiny amounts of a variety of minerals. Some of these trace minerals have specific functions that we can document, but our understanding of their roles in maintaining life and health is really only in its infancy. There are few studies dealing with the trace minerals in human pregnancy, so information is gathered from animal studies and from blood and tissue samples of humans.

Iron, zinc, and iodine are the only trace minerals that have RDA-type recommendations for levels of consumption during pregnancy. Some other trace minerals have tentative recommendations for "safe and adequate" ranges of consumption by adults but none of these tentative recommendations is specific to pregnancy.

Most trace minerals are easily obtained through a varied diet. Unfortunately, some people seem to think that if a little is good, a lot is better. If excessive amounts of the trace minerals are consumed, they may be dangerous to you and your unborn child.

### Pumping Iron

■ *Women who are in their childbearing years are more likely to be deficient in iron than any other nutrient.* Many women, like Janet, enter pregnancy with a deficiency:

"I somehow had the impression that 'iron-poor blood' was a condition that accompanied aging. My lifestyle of work and recreation kept me active from morn to night, and I was seldom sick, so it never occurred to me that I needed more iron. I went to the doctor when I thought I was pregnant. I was delighted to have the pregnancy confirmed and astonished to learn that I had a significant iron deficiency."

This experience is not unusual. Many women do not realize that even if they eat well, iron is lost through menstruation, and that some foods and medications severely impair the absorption and utilization of iron.

During pregnancy, the need for iron is significantly more than the need before pregnancy. The iron normally lost during menstruation is conserved, and you are likely to absorb more iron from the food you eat. Even then, you may not have enough iron to meet both your own and your developing baby's needs. If your pre-pregnancy diet continues without significantly increasing iron intake, you will soon find yourself suffering the symptoms of "iron-poor blood": fatigue, anemia, and infections. Most American physicians favor routine supplementation of iron during pregnancy. Dr. Marilyn Frederiksen, Specialist in Maternal-Fetal Medicine at Prentice Women's Hospital, Chicago, stated, "We see so many pregnant women with significant iron deficiencies that I think iron supplementation should be prescribed for virtually all women during pregnancy."[171]

As the blood volume increases, there is an increase in the amount of iron needed to form red blood cells. Iron is part of the hemoglobin in these cells. It is the hemoglobin in red blood cells that carries oxygen throughout the body. If you reduce iron, you decrease the amount of hemoglobin and thereby reduce the amount of oxygen that can be supplied to cells, subsequently limiting the amount of energy produced. The result is that you feel tired and listless. A reduced hemoglobin-iron partnership in the blood may also put stress on your heart as it must pump harder and harder in an attempt to supply oxygen to cells. During pregnancy, this effort is increased even more to meet the needs of the placenta and the fetus for oxygen.

During the last trimester, the baby is most demanding as it builds iron reserves for the first three to four months after birth. The baby takes what iron it needs, and doesn't pay a lot of attention to its mother's supplies or needs. Twins, who may not be able to gain ample iron stores, and premature babies, whose period of building iron reserves is shortened, may exhibit an iron deficiency during the first months after birth.

Having iron-deficiency anemia is hardly the best way for a woman to enter the demanding period of labor and delivery! Even though the expanded blood volume allows for losses during delivery, a new mother will need all the energy she can muster for the hard work involved during birth and in the weeks after the baby is born.

A curious symptom associated with a low iron intake is *pica*. (Women with normal iron levels have also been known to have this strange craving.) Women with pica eat non-food items such as clay, laundry starch, cornstarch, or paint. Although pica has usually been described in studies of low-income populations, women of all socio-economic groups can exhibit it. Mary had a friend who called her late one night in a panic. "I'm standing in my laundry room eating starch. I feel driven to eat it. What's going on? Am I going crazy?" She was embarrassed to tell her doctor. Sure enough, she had stopped taking her iron supplements and hadn't told the doctor that either. Mary told her to call the doctor in the morning and to start taking her prescribed iron. If she felt that she could not talk to her doctor, then maybe it was time to shop for a doctor instead of a layette. When the iron supplements were re-started, the pica stopped —to everyone's relief.

Some women eat ice cubes (even when not pregnant) to alleviate the discomfort of the gums and tongue that can be caused by iron deficiency. This is one of the few instances where specific deprivations are related to cravings during pregnancy. It represents a condition that could potentially be harmful to your baby.

When the NRC formulated the RDAs, it stated, "The increased requirements during pregnancy cannot be met by the iron content of habitual American diets or by the existing iron stores of many women; therefore, the use of 30 to 60 milligrams supplementary iron is recommended. Iron needs during lactation are not substantially different from those of non-pregnant women, but continued supplementation of the mother for two to three months after parturition [delivery] is advisable to replenish stores depleted by pregnancy."[6]

Supplements do play an important role in meeting needs, but they cannot do it alone. Supplementary iron may not be absorbed as well as dietary iron. Iron supplements marked "ferrous sulfate" and "ferrous fumarate" are reported to be absorbed better than those with iron in forms called "iron phosphate," "iron pyrophosphate," and "iron orthophosphate." Iron supplements must be taken in small, frequent doses because the digestive tract cannot absorb large single doses of iron. This limits both the total amount that can be given and the ease with which it can be taken. Many women admit that they are not diligent in taking their iron pills regularly because iron may cause constipation or indigestion. Taking iron medications with a glass of orange juice or some other source of vitamin C increases its absorption. There is no evidence that slow-release preparations or other forms of iron pills are more effectively absorbed or utilized.[100]

Even good things can be dangerous. Be sure that any iron supplements you take are kept away from small children. Many small children who think that pills are candy have been hospitalized owing to iron poisoning from accidental ingestion of Mom's iron pills. Childproof bottles help, but don't keep iron pills or any other medication on the kitchen counter or any place that children can reach. Lots of people keep vitamin-mineral supplements in the kitchen, but this may invite trouble. If you need a visual reminder to take the pills, put a note on your refrigerator door or bathroom mirror!

■ *Meeting Iron Needs with Food* Getting enough iron is understandably difficult and a lifelong nutritional problem for many women. A number of factors influence the amount of dietary iron absorption.

* If iron-rich foods are consumed along with foods containing *vitamin C*, such as orange juice or tomatoes, the rate of iron absorption will be almost doubled because the vitamin C helps change iron into its most absorbable form.[47] Iron supplements often contain vitamin C to boost their power.
* The *protein* in meat, fish, and poultry (not the protein in milk, cheese, or eggs) enhances both the digestion and absorption of iron, if they are consumed together. For this reason, iron supplements are best consumed before or just after mealtime when you will also be eating protein.[63]
* *Antacid* medications, the kind commonly taken for heartburn or an upset stomach, can reduce acidity, which can interfere with the absorption of iron and other minerals.
* Tea, if consumed with a meal, reduces the amount of iron absorbed by two-thirds.[68]
* *Chelated EDTA*, a food additive, binds iron, inhibiting its absorption. Read labels, and avoid eating foods containing EDTA when you are eating iron-rich foods or taking iron supplements.
* Recent studies at the Univeristy of Kansas reported that *soy protein* may dramatically reduce iron absorption. If you use significant amounts of soy or other vegetable proteins as meat alternatives, you should be aware of this potential

influence on your total iron consumption. If you are a vegetarian, be sure your physician knows. Dietary iron from animal sources is better utilized than iron from vegetable sources, a fact that places vegetarians at risk of developing iron-deficiency anemia.

* *Phytic acid*, found in green leafy vegetables such as spinach, and *oxalic acid*, found in whole grains, bind with iron and other minerals and prevent the body from using the nutrient present in the food itself. However, unless you eat large amounts of oatmeal or spinach three meals a day, these foods are more a help rather than a hindrance to good nutrition.

* Excess *fiber* can reduce absorption of iron, partly because fiber stimulates elimination of foods from the digestive tract. If iron-rich foods are too quickly removed, your body does not have a chance to absorb the iron.

* One of the best ways to increase the amount of iron in your diet is to *cook with old-fashioned cast-iron skillets and kettles* (the black ones, not the enameled ones). Acid-rich foods draw iron into the food. Spaghetti sauce simmered in an iron pot has almost thirty times more iron content than the same sauce cooked in a non-iron container! Some scientists speculate that the increase in anemia is related to the decreased use of iron cookware.[19]

Recently, Mary's dad was found to be anemic and needed some dietary advice. "I told my mother to go to the neighborhood hardware store and buy an old-fashioned cast-iron skillet for daily cooking. She told me a few days later that she had purchased one and that the saleswoman said, 'I didn't know your husband was a doctor.' My mother said that he wasn't a doctor and asked why the saleswoman thought he was. The response was 'Because doctors' wives always buy these pots!' "

Good dietary sources of iron are liver (especially good), red meats, sardines, lima beans, dried fruits and nuts, canned baked beans, prune juice, and blackstrap molasses. *Liver is absolutely the best source of iron.* About 28 percent of Americans' dietary iron is found in enriched and fortified foods, such as macaroni, rice, cornmeal, bread and cereals. Milk, dairy products, and fresh fruits are low in iron. The iron found in dried fruits is a result of absorption of iron from the drying trays into the fruit during the long drying time. It is a variation on the cast-iron skillet trick!

| FOOD SOURCES OF IRON [34] | | |
|---|---|---|
| Food | Portion | Milligrams Iron |
| Calves' liver, fried | 3½ oz. | 14.2 |
| Liverwurst | 3 ounces | 8.7 |
| Chicken livers, cooked | 3½ oz. | 8.5 |
| Prune juice | ¾ cup | 7.4 |
| Ground beef, lean, cooked | 3½ oz. | 3.8 |
| Sardines | 8 medium | 3.5 |
| Pork chop, lean, cooked | 1 medium | 3.5 |
| Sirloin steak, cooked | 3½ oz. | 3.0 |
| Raisins | ½ cup | 2.5 |
| Molasses, blackstrap | 1 Tbsp. | 2.3 |
| Prunes, dried | 4 large | 2.2 |
| Spinach, cooked | ½ cup | 2.0 |
| Farina, enriched, cooked | 1 cup | 2.0 |
| Turnip greens, cooked | 1 cup | 1.8 |
| Chicken, broiled | 3½ oz. | 1.7 |
| Split peas, cooked | ½ cup | 1.5 |
| Apricots, dried | 4 halves | 1.3 |
| Egg | 1 medium | 1.1 |
| Rye bread | 1 slice | 0.8 |
| White bread, enriched | 1 slice | 0.6 |
| White bread, unenriched | 1 slice | 0.2 |
| Dry cereal | 1 cup | Widely varied, many high; read labels |

## Iodine and Fluorine: Added Protection

Iodine is abundant in seawater and in soil adjacent to the sea, but is absent in the inland soils of our country.

Iodine is a component of *thyroxine*, a substance produced by the thyroid gland. This important gland is located at the base of your throat. Your doctor examines the thyroid gland when he examines your neck. *Thyroxine* regulates the rate at which the body uses energy. If iodine levels in the diet are low, the level of thyroxine produced by the thyroid gland falls, energy levels fall, and there is abnormal weight gain. At the same time, the thyroid gland may enlarge, creating a condition called *goiter*. In some areas of the world, where iodine is not readily available from the diet, iodine deficiency can create problems for both mother and baby. Severely iodine-deficient infants can be born with an irreversible mental retardation and abnormal body structure called *cretinism*.

In areas where iodine is not readily available naturally, *iodized salt* is the most reliable source of iodine. It's easy, it's cheap, and only a small amount is needed. Iodine-deficiency goiter was common in certain areas of the United States until iodized salt was introduced in 1924; now iodine-deficiency goiter is very rare in this country.

Some people think *sea salt* is better for them than regular table salt. Not so. True sea salt is too impure to be sold as food. What is sold has very small amounts of minerals as well as sodium and chloride. Natural iodine is lost when the seawater is washed to remove impurities.[19] Some "sea salts" have iodine added, in the same way regular table salt does.

In the United States, ample iodine is available through dietary sources, including iodized salt, to meet the RDA of 175 micrograms a day. Currently, the American food supply contains plentiful iodine and there is no evidence that pregnant women in the United States need worry about meeting their own or baby's needs.

You should be cautious about taking iodine-containing asthma medications when you are pregnant. The very large doses of iodine that some of these medications contain could create an iodine imbalance and thyroid-gland problems in the newborn.

*Fluorine* (or *fluoride*, which is a form of fluorine) is an important mineral with a starring role in public controversy. Adding it to the public water supply has been a continuing source of political debate. Those who favor its addition point to impressive statistics showing a reduction in tooth decay in areas with flouridated water. Opponents say that chemicals added to water violate individual rights and that those who want it can get it from sources other than the community water supply. Because large amounts can be poisonous, some see it as life-threatening. There is no reliable research to justify these fears.

*Fluorine bonds calcium and phosphorus in bones and teeth to make a structure that is strong and teeth that are resistant to decay.* Tooth decay has been reduced by more than 50 percent in communities that have added fluoride to water at the low level of one part per million (one ppm).[46] One part per million is a very, very tiny amount—like a drop of water in a swimming pool or a drop of vermouth in a tank car of gin.

Fluoride is naturally present in some water, usually well water, and in amounts in excess of one ppm in some places. Excessive fluoride can cause discolored spots on teeth, which, while it isn't physically harmful, isn't cosmetically desirable.

Whether the maternal intake of fluoride during pregnancy influences a child's later resistance to tooth decay has not been determined.[18] Babies drink the same water their mother did and we cannot tell *when* the positive effect influences teeth. We do know that fluoride plays an important role in bone formation and in the depositing of calcium into teeth, which begins in the fifth month of pregnancy. If you live in an area that does not have fluoridated water, ask your dentist about fluoride treatments for you and your family. Some physicians recommend that pregnant women take 1 milligram of fluoride per day throughout pregnancy if they are not drinking water that has been fluoridated—whether because they live in an area that does not have fluoridated water, or they drink milk and juice and other beverages in place of fluoridated water from the tap.

### Is It True What They Say about Oysters?

The very best dietary source of *zinc* is oysters. The connection between zinc and sexuality, no doubt, accounts for the "sexy" reputation enjoyed by oysters. Does this mean that if you eat Atlantic oysters, which have eight times more zinc than Pacific oysters, you will be sexier? Although severe zinc deficiencies may result in retarded sexual growth, and it has been shown that zinc can be used to treat impotency of men who lose zinc through kidney dialysis, zinc cannot cure general impotence. Since impotency is not a problem associated with pregnancy, this may not be of interest to you, but may make eating oysters more enjoyable and can certainly add to the table conversation.

You are going to hear a lot about zinc in the years ahead. Scientific understanding of its role in human growth and development has only just begun. Zinc is important to digestion, metabolism, breathing, wound healing, and maintaining skin and hair. Zinc deficiency has been associated with retarded growth, delayed sexual maturity, skin rashes, and poor appetite.[18] New evidence is continually being published that suggests the great influence of zinc on fetal development. Animal studies indicate that the fetus requires dietary zinc because the mother does not release zinc from her own body tissues to meet the needs of the fetus.[1] There is no human body storage depot of zinc, so a good dietary intake seems particularly important.

Many zinc experiments are done with laboratory test animals. In recent reports, the offspring of rats who were deprived of zinc during the later third of pregnancy demonstrated severe fetal growth retardation, missing limbs, and decreased brain growth.[1] Zinc is essential for protein synthesis and brain growth. Retarded brain growth may explain the outcome of tests showing that the offspring of zinc-deprived monkeys had behavioral problems.

How much zinc the pregnant woman needs has not been firmly established, but the National Research Council has set 20 milligrams as the RDA. This assumes adequate protein from animal sources. It may not be enough for some women (especially vegetarians) who rely heavily on whole grains in their diet. Zinc, like iron, can be bound by the phytates in whole grains, reducing absorption.

Recent evidence suggests that many Americans may not be getting enough zinc. Much of the naturally available zinc in foods is removed during processing—a fact that has led some researchers at the University of Colorado Medical Center to recommend fortification of cereals with zinc.

Since content is not generally listed on labels, you should

become aware of food sources of zinc and include them in your diet. A good varied diet that does not overly rely on processed foods should provide enough zinc.

Zinc toxicity is rare, though megadoses are becoming more common as zinc gains popularity as a self-help remedy for a variety of problems. It is widely promoted in health food stores as a dietary supplement, both alone and in combination with various vitamins and minerals. Premature and stillborn births have recently been reported among women who took large doses of supplementary zinc during the third trimester of pregnancy.[1] Infants born to mothers who took megadoses of zinc have a greatly increased incidence of birth defects.[100]

| GOOD SOURCES OF ZINC [34] | | |
|---|---|---|
| Daily need in pregnancy—20 milligrams | | |
| Food | Portion | Milligrams Zinc |
| Oysters, Atlantic, raw or frozen | 3 oz. | 63.0 |
| Oysters, Pacific, raw or frozen | 3 oz. | 7.6 |
| Calves' liver, cooked | 3 oz. | 5.3 |
| Beef, lean, cooked | 3 oz. | 5.1 |
| Lamb, lean, cooked | 3 oz. | 4.0 |
| Crabmeat | ½ cup | 3.4 |
| Blackeye peas, cooked | ½ cup | 3.4 |
| Pork loin, cooked | 3 oz. | 2.6 |
| Chicken, leg and thigh meat | 3 oz. | 2.4 |
| Shrimp, canned | ½ cup | 1.4 |
| Yogurt, plain | 1 cup | 1.1 |
| Potato, baked with skin | 1 medium | 1.0 |
| Tuna, oil-packed, drained | 3 oz. | .9 |
| Lima beans, cooked | ½ cup | .9 |
| Peas, green, cooked | ½ cup | .9 |
| Whitefish, broiled | 3 oz. | .9 |
| Whole milk | 1 cup | .9 |
| Macaroni, cooked | 1 cup | .7 |
| Egg | 1 large | .5 |
| Cottage cheese, creamed | ½ cup | .5 |
| Avocado | ½ medium | .5 |

### Copper: A Hidden Treasure?

As of 1980, there was no RDA for copper, but the "estimated and adequate" safe range for healthy adults was established at 2 to 3 milligrams per day. There is no range recommended specifically for pregnancy. When you know that copper levels in the blood of pregnant women are 2½ times higher than in non-pregnant women, you can be pretty sure there is a reason![18] That reason, however, is not yet fully understood.

What we do know is that copper plays a vital role in the storage and release of iron to form hemoglobin, so adequate copper is especially important during the first months of pregnancy when iron is needed for expanding blood volume, and also throughout pregnancy to help prevent anemia.

A list of copper functions sounds like a home repair manual! Copper tubing and wires and insulators run to nerves and bones and skin and hair. On the basis of weight, the brain is the most concentrated site of copper. During the mother's pregnancy, the fetus builds up stores of copper in its liver to sustain it during the first two to three months after birth.[75]

Copper deficiencies are rare because copper is widely available in foods. The best sources are whole grains, shellfish, liver and kidney, raisins, nuts, peas and beans, and fresh fruits and vegetables. Copper can be dangerous if taken in high doses. Consistently eating acid foods, such as tomatoes, cooked in unlined copper pots could cause possible toxicity.

### More Trace Minerals

There are other trace minerals that have been shown to be essential to animal life, but little is known about their functions. The fact that they have so recently been identified as necessary is an indication that many more may be identified in the future.

The following chart gives information on chromium, cobalt, manganese, and selenium. Other minerals believed to be essential for animal life include molybdenum, nickel, vanadium, tin, and silicon. Little is known about these, and virtually nothing in relation to human pregnancy. We must wait for further scientific research to tell us about them.

The following chart shows why "Eat a variety of foods" is important advice.

# ESSENTIAL TRACE ELEMENTS

|  | Chromium | Cobalt |
|---|---|---|
| Functions | Acts with insulin, necessary for glucose utilization | Part of Vitamin $B_{12}$ |
| Food Sources | Meat, poultry, brewer's yeast, whole grains, cereals, liver, milk, cheese | Animal foods: meat, liver, milk, eggs, dairy products, poultry, fish |
| Comments | Chromium can be lost in food processing. Chromium is being studied in relation to diabetes mellitus. | Strict vegetarians may have difficulty meeting needs, others meet needs easily. |

|  | Manganese | Selenium |
|---|---|---|
| Functions | Necessary for normal bone and tendon structure | Anti-oxidant |
|  |  | Related to vitamin E |
|  | Necessary for release of energy from fats and glucose |  |
|  | Aids in protein metabolism |  |
|  | Affects central nervous system |  |
| Food Sources | Bran, cereals, nuts, peas and beans, coffee, tea | Seafood, meat, liver, poultry, asparagus, mushrooms, milk, egg yolk |
| Comments | An expert panel of Food and Drug Administration has stated that manganese can be dangerous when taken in high doses. | The most toxic of the essential nutrients. |
|  | Human deficiency unknown. Deficiencies in animals cause growth defects and abnormal nervous systems. | Excesses can cause death in animals. |

## Trace Mineral Supplements

Virtually all the known minerals are available in foods; the unknown ones, no doubt, are there too. Throughout human history, we have eaten foods, not food supplements. It seems reasonable to assume, therefore, that foods, and not megadoses of vitamins or minerals, will continue to provide the necessary nutrients.

*Overdoses of minerals can be very dangerous.* Bone meal and dolomite, taken for extra calcium, often contain contaminants that might cause lead poisoning. Too much calcium, even if pure, can cause drowsiness and reduce the absorption of iron, zinc, and manganese. Some minerals work in balance with others, so too much of one can interfere with utilization of another. Large doses of most trace minerals—copper, fluorine, selenium, manganese, and molybdenum—could poison you. Excesses of zinc are linked to everything from nausea to premature birth. *All of these potential dangers are from supplements, not from foods.* You cannot overdose on peas, nuts, or any other food. Advice given by friends or relatives to take supplements, though well-meaning, may jeopardize your health or your baby's. *Do not take any vitamin or mineral supplement unless it is prescribed by your doctor—and then, only in the amounts prescribed.*

# 7.
# Making
# Food Choices:
# A Nutritional
# Game Plan

## QUICK QUIZ

■ *Step 1:*

Write down on a piece of paper all the food that you ate yesterday from the time you woke up until you went to sleep. Be sure to include snacks and beverages, even water.

■ *Step 2:*

Now look at each of the foods you listed and put one mark for each item you ate in the groups we have listed where it best fits. Give one mark for a regular-size portion, for instance, a salad would get one mark for raw vegetable, even if it had lettuce, tomatoes, and cucumbers. Total the number of servings from each group.

|          | *Foods*                        | *Your Intake* |
|----------|--------------------------------|---------------|
| Group 1: | Milk (also credit Group 6)     |               |
|          | Yogurt                         |               |
|          | Cheese                         |               |
|          | Ice cream                      |               |
|          | Puddings, custard              |               |
|          | Other dairy products           |               |
|          |                                | Total for day _____ |

|  | *Foods* | *Your Intake* |
|---|---|---|

**Group 2:** Fresh fruit juice (also credit Group 6)
Canned fruit
Raw vegetable or salad
Dried fruit
Other fruits or vegetables

Total for day _____

**Group 3:** Bread, roll, etc.
Cereal
Grain, rice
Noodles, pasta

Total for day _____

**Group 4:** Meat
Fish or poultry
Dried beans or peas
Nuts
Eggs
Other protein foods

Total for day _____

**Group 5:** Sugar
Sweets, candy
Salad dressing
Butter or margarine
Cream
Fried food (Also credit the food category; i.e., fried chicken also counts one mark for poultry.)

Total for day _____

**Group 6:** Water, 1 glass
Milk (also credit Group 1)
Fruit juice (also credit Group 2)
Coffee or tea
Soda pop
Other beverages

Total for day _____

How many glasses of beer, wine, liquor or other beverages containing alcohol did you have yesterday? _____ Do you drink more on weekends?
_____
List foods that do not fit any of the above groups.

■ *Step 3:*

Sit down, put your feet up, and read this chapter.

■ *Step 4:*

Now, evaluate yesterday's food intake on the basis of what you need. How close were you to the recommended number of servings for each group listed on page 124? Are there whole groups of foods you do not eat that could be depriving you of necessary nutrients? What can you do to improve your diet tomorrow?

In this chapter, we are going to move our discussion to the supermarket, the cafeteria, the restaurant, the dinner party, the kitchen—to the places where you make food choices.

You will need to draw up a "diet game plan" to assess your strengths and weaknesses, and make substitutions where necessary. Every day you can work at making good food choices, guided by this book. The goal of a healthier baby is worth the effort.

Mary comments: "Years of experience in dietary counseling have convinced me that diet plans must be individualized. There are diets that call for specific foods on a schedule. Many of these diets are very nutritious—on paper. But if the foods listed never make it to your mouth, the diet cannot be nutritious for you or your baby. What good is it to tell you to eat something you do not like, do not know how to prepare, or cannot afford to buy?"

## A Diet That Works

* is based on your habits, preferences, and needs,
* provides information so that you can make rational food choices based on fact rather than pickles-and-ice-cream stories, and
* gives you a gentle push in the right direction by giving you the straight scoop about what good eating can do, and warnings about potential dangers.

Many factors influence which foods you choose to eat: ethnic background, income, ease of preparation, cooking skills and equipment, others in your family, how often you eat away from home, taste preferences.

Pregnancy brings a new awareness to the choices you make. You may decide to include some foods you have not eaten regularly before. There may also be unexpected and unexplained additions.

There are few instances where there is a physiological reason for a specific craving during pregnancy. Some women crave non-food substances such as cornstarch or ice, which may be linked to an iron deficiency (see Chapter 6), and there is evidence of salt cravings arising from a deficiency.

As for pickles and ice cream, the only explanation may be that they bring *comfort* and *joy*—pretty essential "nutrients" in our thinking! Mary had gourmet food cravings when she was pregnant; she assures us they were very real! "I had no food cravings during my previous pregnancy, but with Leslie, I craved gorgonzola cheese and figs in the evening. I do not remember ever eating these foods before I became pregnant, much less together. Several years later, while traveling in Italy, I learned that it is a classic Italian combination. Leslie knew that before birth."

### Hey, Dad! You're Eating for Two, Too

Having a baby is a family affair. One of the most significant ways a father can become involved is to take an active and supportive role in the mother's prenatal diet. There's a lot to learn about all the nutrients and their role in pregnancy. Prospective parents can read this book together and discuss its implications for their meal planning. If dietary changes are necessary, it will be easier to do it together. *Pregnancy is a good time to improve the eating patterns of the entire family.* With few exceptions, what's good for mother and baby during pregnancy will be good for everyone in the family. Those few exceptions have been pointed out in previous chapters: It may be wise for other family members to limit foods rich in cholesterol and saturated fat and to reduce their intake of salt.

## A FATHER'S GUIDE TO THE CARE AND FEEDING OF PREGNANT WOMEN

* Encourage Mom to seek early prenatal care. Stay with other children if necessary, or go with her if she wants you to be there. Help her decide on an obstetrician or family physician who has time to answer questions about health concerns including nutrition.
* Encourage regular eating patterns. This may mean that you will end up being responsible for preparing or bringing home some of the meals. Play "milkman." Make sure there's a quart a day (or its equivalent) exclusively for Mom.
* Remind Mom to take her vitamin-mineral supplements, if they are prescribed.
* Bring home beautiful fresh fruits and vegetables along with an occasional bouquet of flowers.
* Help plan and shop for nutritious foods. Be willing to try new foods along with Mom.
* If "morning sickness" strikes, remember, you are partially responsible! Do what you can by providing moral support, soda crackers, or whatever Mom wants, with love and understanding. Do not expect her to make your breakfast!
* When eating out, remind Mom to order foods that are good for her that might not be prepared at home. How about a chopped liver appetizer or calves' liver and onions? Many restaurants prepare liver well and it is a good source of almost every nutrient.

### Six Food Groups

To help you select foods that will provide the nutrients you need, we have divided foods into groups, and suggested the number of selections you need to make from each group in order to have a balanced diet. *A balanced diet is one that provides all of the essential nutrients within a reasonable calorie limit from a variety of foods.*

In school, you may have learned about the *basic four* food groups. We have expanded this to *six food groups*. The added groups help you to meet your need for water and other liquids and to choose fats and sugars to make your food tasty and enjoyable. The food groups are:

1. Milk and dairy products
2. Fruits and vegetables
3. Breads and cereals
4. Protein foods
5. Fats and sugars
6. Water and other liquids

Your needs during pregnancy are different from those of children or adult men. The chart below shows the recommended number of servings for you and other members of your family.

A plus (+) means "or more." One serving meets the basic requirement, but additional servings are good sources of extra nutrients and calories you need during pregnancy.

| DAILY FOOD GUIDE | | | |
|---|---|---|---|
| | Pregnant Women | Non-Pregnant Women | Men | Children |
| Milk and dairy products | 4+ | 2+ | 2+ | 2–3+ |
| Fruits and vegetables (Total) Including: | 5+ | 4+ | 4+ | 4+ |
| Vitamin-C rich | 1+ | 1 | 1 | 1 |
| Deep green, yellow or orange | 2 | At least 3 times a week | At least 3 times a week | At least 3 times a week |
| Other | 2+ | 2+ | 2+ | 2+ |
| Breads and cereals | 4+ | 4+ | 4+ | 4+ |
| Protein foods | 3 | 2 | 2 | 2 |
| Fats and sugars | 2 Tbsp. margarine or oil | As necessary for added calories | | |
| Water, other liquids | 8+ | 6–8 | 6–8 | 6–8 |

### Translating Nutrients into Foods

In the previous chapters, we have given you more information than you probably want to know about nutrients. For each of the nutrients, there was a list of good food sources. You may have noticed that some foods appear on a number of different lists. These foods have a *high nutrient density*.

Nutrient density is calculated by giving pluses for the positive nutritional content in a food, and minuses for added sugar, salt, cholesterol, or saturated fat content. The following charts divide the foods of each group into the *Best Choices* and *Other Choices* based on the nutrient density of the food.

| | |
|---|---|
| Best Choices | The best providers of the nutrients without significant extra calories from sugar or fat. If you are having a problem controlling your weight, make almost all of your food choices from this group. |
| Other Choices | These foods count as servings, but they have either<br>1. smaller amounts of key nutrients, or<br>2. added sugar and fat. |

### 1. Milk and Dairy Products

*Four or more servings are needed each day.*

---

**ONE SERVING**

1 cup of milk or yogurt
1½ oz. hard cheese, such as Cheddar
1½ cups soft cheese, such as cottage cheese

---

Some of the foods you might expect to find listed here are not. Butter, cream, and coffee lighteners all have lots of fat, and are low in calcium, phosphorus, protein, riboflavin, and other nutrients provided by this group. Therefore, they don't count as milk servings, they count as fats.

Ice cream (with or without pickles) can be a part of a

nutritious diet, but keep in mind that it takes two cups of ice cream, with a whopping 556 calories, to get the same amount of calcium as a glass of skim milk, which comes in at 90 calories!

Although we look to milk to meet calcium needs, milk also provides an inexpensive source of complete protein. Instant non-fat dry milk (dry skim milk) is a particularly economical source of many nutrients. If you mix it and refrigerate it for a few hours, the flavor is improved. Some women like to mix about a cup of whole milk in a quart of reconstituted dry milk for do-it-yourself 1 percent low-fat milk.

| Best Choices | Other Choices |
| --- | --- |
| Lowfat, skim milk | Flavored yogurt |
| 1%- or 2%-fat milk | Chocolate milk |
| Buttermilk | Milkshake |
| Whole milk | Ice milk |
| Cheeses (Cheddar, Swiss, Muenster, etc.) | Ice cream |
| Cottage cheese | Frozen yogurt |
| Plain yogurt | Pudding |
| Nonfat dry milk | Custard |
| Evaporated milk | Cheesecake |
| Eggnog | Creamed soup |

## 2. Fruits and Vegetables

*Choose five or more servings of fruits and vegetables each day. At least two of these servings should be fresh fruit or raw vegetables.*

### ONE SERVING

1 cup raw fruit or vegetable
¾ cup cooked fruit or vegetable
½ cup juice
1 medium size piece of fruit or vegetable, for example, one apple

This group supplies important vitamins, including vitamins A and C and folacin, as well as minerals and fiber. Because this food group must supply several key nutrients, there are *Best Choices* listings for both vitamins A and C.

Some fruits and vegetables—cantaloupe and broccoli, for example—appear in both of the *Best Choices* columns. If you eat one of these foods, you get a nutritional double whammy, but you still need a *total* of at least five servings of fruits and vegetables. These are foods with very high nutrient density.

The column labeled *Second-Best Choices* contains foods that are not as high in the nutrient density as the foods in the first two columns, but they do contribute to the total vitamins, minerals, and fiber that you need each day, and provide variety and interest.

The *Other Choices* are fruit and vegetables prepared with fat or sugar. Limit your selections from this group (unless you need to gain weight), and try to balance out their higher calorie content by making other prudent food choices during the day.

## BEST CHOICES

|  | *Vitamin C-Rich* | *Deep Green, Yellow, or Orange (Vitamin A)* |  |
|---|---|---|---|
| *Fruits* | Acerola cherry | Apricot |  |
|  | Cantaloupe | Cantaloupe |  |
|  | Grapefruit | Mango |  |
|  | Guava | Papaya |  |
|  | Lemon | Pumpkin |  |
|  | Mango |  |  |
|  | Orange |  |  |
|  | Papaya |  |  |
|  | Strawberries | *Second-Best Choices* |  |
|  | Tangerine |  |  |
|  |  | Apple | Honeydew melon |
|  |  | Avocado | Nectarine |
|  |  | Banana | Peach |
|  |  | Blackberries | Pear |
|  |  | Blueberries | Persimmon |
|  |  | Boysenberries | Pineapple |
|  |  | Casaba melon | Plum |
|  |  | Cherries | Plantain |
|  |  | Currants | Prunes |
|  |  | Dates | Raisins |
|  |  | Dried fruit | Raspberries |
|  |  | Figs | Rhubarb |
|  |  | Grapes | Watermelon |

# BEST CHOICES *(cont.)*

|  | Vitamin C-Rich | Deep Green, Yellow, or Orange (Vitamin A) | Second-Best Choices |
|---|---|---|---|
| *Juices* | Cranberry (fortified with vitamin C) Orange Tangerine Tomato Vegetable juice cocktail | | Apple juice or cider Grape Pineapple Prune |
| *Vegetables* | Broccoli Brussels sprouts Cabbage Cauliflower Kale Green pepper Rutabaga Sweet potato Swiss chard Tomato | Beet greens Broccoli Brussels sprouts Carrot Chicory Collard greens Dandelion greens Escarole Kale Lettuce Mixed vegetables Mustard greens Spinach Sweet potato Swiss chard Winter squash (acorn, hubbard, butternut) | Alfafa sprouts Artichoke Asparagus Beans (kidney, garbanzo, green beans, limas, wax beans, bean sprouts) Beets Celery Corn Cucumber Eggplant Kohlrabi Leeks Mushrooms Okra Onions Parsnip Peas Potato Radishes Scallions Summer squash Turnips Yams |

## OTHER CHOICES

| | |
|---|---|
| *Fruits* | Applesauce |
| | Fruits canned in syrup |
| | Candied fruits |
| | Fruit drinks (orange drink, etc.) |
| | Fruit nectars (apricot, pear, etc.) |
| | Lemonade |
| | Fruit pies, cobblers, or crisps |
| | |
| *Vegetables* | Deep-fried vegetables |
| | Potato chips, potato sticks, potato salad |
| | Pumpkin or sweet-potato pie |
| | Salads with excessive dressing |
| | Sauerkraut |
| | Vegetables in cream sauce |
| | Vegetables frozen in sauces |

## 3. Breads and Cereals

*Choose four or more servings from this group each day.*

### ONE SERVING

1 slice bread
1 muffin, bagel, tortilla
½ English muffin or bun
½–¾ cup cooked cereal
¾–1 cup (1 ounce) ready-to-eat cereal
½–¾ cup rice, noodles, spaghetti, grits
4–8 crackers, depending on size

Breads and cereals are made from grains. *Whole-grain breads* are made from whole kernels that have been ground into flour. Breads and cereals made from rye or whole-wheat flour are whole-grain products.

Other types of breads and cereals are made from more highly processed flours. In milling, the *bran*, which is the outer covering of the kernel of wheat, and the *germ*, which is the

| Restored: | Vitamins and minerals are returned to the food at the same level as the original food. |
| Enriched: | Three vitamins and one mineral that were removed in processing are returned at the levels determined by food laws. These levels are slightly higher than what was removed. Most flour and many breads are enriched. |
| Fortified: | Vitamins, minerals, and sometimes protein that were not in the original food are added as the food is processed, prior to packaging. Many breakfast cereals are fortified. |

innermost part, are removed. The result of such milling is white flour. Many vitamins and minerals are lost when the bran and germ are removed. Flour and other foods can be treated to add nutrients; they can be *restored, fortified,* or *enriched.* The label will tell you what has been done.

If you regularly eat a fortified cereal, in addition to taking a prenatal multivitamin, be sure to tell your doctor. Some fortified cereals contain as much as 100 percent of the RDA for specific nutrients, so it may be desirable to omit the balanced prenatal supplement and take only folacin and iron to avoid oversupplementation.

The *Best Choices* list for Breads and Cereals is divided into whole-grain and enriched/restored/fortified foods.

Although whole-grain bread has a long list of pluses, it also contains phytic acid, which can reduce the absorption of several minerals. Nonetheless, the benefits far outweigh this disadvantage and whole-grain bread should be included in your diet every day.

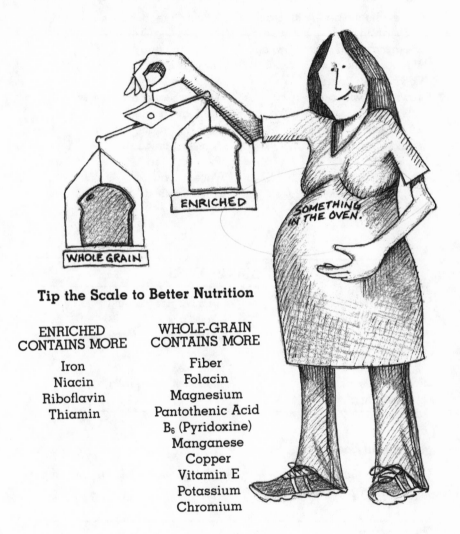

## Tip the Scale to Better Nutrition

ENRICHED
CONTAINS MORE

Iron
Niacin
Riboflavin
Thiamin

WHOLE-GRAIN
CONTAINS MORE

Fiber
Folacin
Magnesium
Pantothenic Acid
$B_6$ (Pyridoxine)
Manganese
Copper
Vitamin E
Potassium
Chromium

## BEST CHOICES

*Whole Grain*

Whole-wheat bread, rolls, crackers
Whole-grain cereals, hot or ready-
    to-eat (oatmeal), cracked wheat,
    shredded wheat, etc.)
Wheat germ
Brown rice, wild rice
Millet, barley
Cornbread, or corn muffins
Tortilla
Whole-wheat pita
Rye bread or crackers
Pumpernickel bread
Popcorn, unbuttered

*Enriched/Restored/Fortified*

Enriched bread, rolls, buns
Enriched biscuits
English muffins
Corn grits, farina
White rice
Puffed wheat or rice, restored
Mixed-grain cereals
Pasta, macaroni, noodles
Crackers, bread sticks
Bagel, bialy roll
White pita bread
Cereals without excessive sugar

## OTHER CHOICES

White breads, not enriched
Buttered popcorn
Graham crackers
Granola
Highly sugared cereals
Fruit breads, nut breads
Bread stuffing

Bread or rice pudding
Croissants
Doughnuts, sweet rolls
Cookies
Pancakes, waffles
Macaroni, pasta salads

### 4. Protein Foods

*You need a source of complete protein at each meal—or three servings of high-quality protein food, besides milk, each day.*

### ONE SERVING

3 oz. cooked lean meat, poultry, or fish
2 eggs
1½ cups cooked dry peas, beans,
    soybeans, or lentils

4 Tbsp. peanut butter
1–1½ cups nuts, sesame seeds,
    or sunflower seeds
8 ounces tofu (soybean curd)

## BEST CHOICES

*Animal*

Liver, organ meats
Lean beef, lamb, pork, veal
Chicken
Turkey
Fish
Shellfish (shrimp, oysters, lobster, crab)
Eggs
Turkey franks, chicken franks, turkey ham
Cornish game hens

*Vegetable*

Blackeye peas
Garbanzo beans
Kidney (pinto) beans
Lentils
Lima beans
Pea beans
Split peas
Soybeans
Textured vegetable protein (TVP)
Tofu

## OTHER CHOICES

Most of these choices are high in fat and calories, but they also provide valuable protein. Generally, they contain more calories from fat than from protein.

*Animal*

Sausages, frankfurters
Bologna, salami, cold cuts
Spareribs and other fatty cuts of pork
Breaded fish sticks
Corned beef, shortribs, and fatty cuts of beef

Goose
Duck
Fried meats
Fried chicken
Fried fish

*Vegetable*

Nuts
Peanut butter
Sesame seeds
Sunflower seeds

Some people limit egg consumption because egg yolks contain cholesterol, but we encourage pregnant women to eat some eggs because they are a quick, easy, economical source of protein and other key nutrients. However, the American Heart Association and the Dietary Guidelines for the United States[162] suggest that it would be prudent for the general population to limit their consumption of eggs and other sources of cholesterol. You may want to have more eggs than other family members.

A vegetarian who eats no poultry or fish, but consumes a wide range of grains, legumes, nuts, fruits, vegetables, and dairy products, can have a nutritionally adequate diet for her own and her baby's needs. For vegetarians, one egg, some cheese, and four glasses of milk (or the equivalent in cheese) each day is good insurance that protein needs will be met.

Vegetarians who do not eat eggs or use other dairy products have a more difficult time meeting protein needs. If grains and vegetables are chosen in the correct combinations, protein needs can be met, although supplementary vitamins and minerals will be required. Again, we emphasize that *it is important for the vegetarian mother-to-be to consume adequate calories, so that the protein she eats will not be used to meet energy needs.*

### 5. Fats and Oils; Sugars and Sweets

This category primarily provides calories to the diet since you need only two tablespoons of oil each day during pregnancy. A little bit of butter or margarine may help the green beans go down, but very often, the little bit gets to be a lot. Next time you stand in line at the salad bar, think about this: Americans consume approximately 345 million gallons of salad dressing a year—that's a little more than one quart per person per week, at sixty to eighty calories *per tablespoon.*[103] But who stops at one tablespoon?

## FOODS WITH DIFFERENT FAT LEVELS

|  | Portion | Grams Fat | Calories |
|---|---|---|---|
| Potatoes |  |  |  |
| Plain, boiled | 1 medium | .1 | 76 |
| Baked | 2½" diameter | .1 | 95 |
| with sour cream | 2 Tbsp. | 6 | 147 |
| with butter or margarine | 1 Tbsp. | 12 | 203 |
| French fries | ½ cup | 12 | 228 |
| Eggs |  |  |  |
| Boiled or poached | 1 medium | 6 | 78 |
| Fried in 1 tsp. margarine | 1 medium | 9 | 108 |
| Toast (whole-wheat) | 1 slice | 1 | 55 |
| with butter or margarine | 1 tsp. | 5 | 91 |
| Chicken |  |  |  |
| Broiled, breast | 3½ oz. | 4 | 166 |
| Fried, breast | 3½ oz. | 12 | 232 |

The way food is prepared and seasoned can make a big difference in the amount of fat—and calories—you add to your diet. The same is true of sugar. How much sugar do you add to your breakfast cereal? Do you choose an apple (87 calories) or apple pie (410 calories)? We aren't suggesting cutting out apple pie entirely, just using the high-sugar, high-fat alternative in moderation.

|  | BEST CHOICES | OTHER CHOICES |
| --- | --- | --- |
| Fats and Oils: | *Moderate Amounts of:* | |
| | Butter | Cream cheese |
| | Margarine | Fried foods |
| | Mayonnaise | Gravy |
| | Salad dressings | Lard |
| | Sour half and half | Potato chips, corn chips |
| | Vegetable oil, salad oil | Sour cream |
| Sugar and Sweets: | *Moderate Amounts of:* | |
| | Honey | Cake |
| | Preserves, jam | Candy |
| | Maple syrup | Coffeecake |
| | Molasses | Cookies |
| | Sugar | Doughnuts |
| | Sugar in fruit-flavored | Flavored gelatin |
| | yogurt, frozen yogurt, | Pastry |
| | ice milk, ice cream | Pie |
| | | Popsicles |
| | | Sherbet |
| | | Sweet rolls |

*You do not have to give up your favorite foods—enjoy them in reasonable amounts, and do not overdo on any given day.*

* Use two tablespoons of dressing on your salad, not a quarter-cup.
* Eat two cookies with your milk instead of six.
* Choose a regular cereal and add one or two teaspoons of sugar instead of eating super-sweetened ready-to-eat cereal.
* Drink real fruit juice instead of sweetened fruit drinks that are fruit-flavored sugar water.

* Make carrot cake instead of chocolate cake.
* On the day you have pie for lunch, eat a piece of fruit for dessert after dinner.
 Choose rice pudding instead of fruit-flavored gelatin for dessert.
* Try a squeeze of lemon on your fish instead of tartar sauce.

## 6. Water and Other Liquids

The nutrient most vital to human life is a beverage that is usually free, is readily available, requires no preparation, and has no calories! If it were being advertised, you would no doubt recognize what has just been described. Unfortunately, you hear much more about liquid competitors, which may have won a more prominent place in your diet than the no-frills product that comes straight from the tap: WATER. *Few people consciously include water in their diet. You rarely think of it, unless you are deprived of it, yet it is an essential nutrient that must be frequently replenished to sustain life.*

More than half of your body—ten to twelve gallons—is water. It assists in absorption, digestion, lubrication, waste removal, and temperature maintenance. Two-and-a-half to three quarts are lost each day, primarily through urination and perspiration. This must be replaced to keep the system running smoothly.

During pregnancy, you need even more water to maintain your expanded blood supply. Intake must be increased to eight or more glasses each day. If you are not accustomed to consuming glasses of water, this may sound impossible. But there is water in many other liquids that help meet this need. If you drink four 8-ounce glasses of milk and a glass of juice, you have about five glasses already and only need three glasses of water. Some additional liquid comes from "solid food." Fruits and vegetables contain over 90 percent water, and even meat is about 50 percent water.

Many women are faced with a real "drinking problem" during pregnancy. They may not be regular milk drinkers and drinking four glasses a day is difficult. Water intake may be limited to a few sips from a drinking fountain. Alcoholic and caffeine-containing beverages are questionable choices. Their main beverage may be soft drinks (soda pop), which have few nutritionally redeeming qualities. *Soft drinks* are loaded with sugar; have many calories; add extra phosphorus, which may interfere with calcium usage; and are acidic, contributing to tooth decay. If you normally drink soft drinks, try to reduce the amount you drink and substitute more nutritious beverages.

In our country, consumption of soft drinks has nearly quadrupled since 1960, and both coffee and beer are consumed in greater quantities than milk.[124] *Choosing beverages that provide water and contribute nutrients to meet the needs of pregnancy without subjecting your baby to unnecessary dangers may be one of the greatest challenges to your current dietary patterns.*

Keep in mind that *fluoridated water* supplies the mineral fluorine needed for developing bones and teeth. If you meet your liquid needs from milk, juice, and soft drinks, and are not drinking water or beverages made from tap water, you may not be getting the fluorine that you and the baby need.

It is considered quite fashionable these days to order bottled *mineral water* with fresh lime or lemon in place of a cocktail. Although it is called mineral water, it is not particularly high in minerals. Dr. Walter Mertz of the Department of Agriculture recently said, "People may like the little bubbles dancing in their glass, but bottled water is not a bit more healthy than tap water."[90] While it is not more healthful, it is not less healthful, either. It is just a different and popular form. In 1980, 380 million gallons of mineral water were sold in the United States.[90]

Most hosts and hostesses thoughtfully provide alternatives for their guests who choose not to drink alcoholic beverages. You may be familiar with the Bloody Mary Cocktail, tomato juice mixed with vodka. A better choice during pregnancy would be the nonalcoholic "Virgin Mary"; or try the "Mother Mary"—the perfect drink for the mother-to-be: 8 ounces of cold, refreshing water on the rocks.

### Multi-Category Foods

A number of popular foods do not appear on the food group lists because they include foods from more than one

## WHAT WILL YOU HAVE TO DRINK?

| Beverage | Amount | Calories | Nutrients | Comment |
|---|---|---|---|---|
| Tap water | 8 oz. (1 cup) | 0 | Fluorine Few trace minerals | None |
| Club soda | 8 oz. | 0 | Sodium | Mother Nature with bubbles. Expensive, tasty water. |
| Tomato juice, canned | 8 oz. | 48 | Vitamin A Vitamin C B vitamins Iron | Aids absorption of iron and other nutrients. |
| Coffee (no cream or sugar) | 8 oz. | 2 | Phosphorus | Caffeine safety questioned during pregnancy.* May act as a diuretic, and remove water from the body. |
| Tea | 8 oz. | 2 | None | Caffeine safety questioned during pregnancy. May act as a diuretic, and remove water from the body. Herb teas (no caffeine) may contain naturally toxic substances. Tea interferes with iron absorption. |
| Milk | 8 oz. | Skim: 90 2%: 120 Whole: 160 | Protein Calcium Phosphorus Riboflavin Vitamins A, D Other vitamins and minerals | Problem only to those who are milk-intolerant. |

## WHAT WILL YOU HAVE TO DRINK? *(cont.)*

| Beverage | Amount | Calories | Nutrients | Comment |
|---|---|---|---|---|
| Orange juice | 8 oz. | 111 | Vitamin C<br>Potassium<br>Vitamin A | Aids absorption of iron and other nutrients. |
| Diet soda pop | 12 oz. | 1 | Sodium | Potential danger from non-nutritive sweetner. May contain caffeine.* |
| Cola drink | 12 oz. | 144 | 9 teaspoons sugar<br>Phosphorus | High sugar content. Caffeine in cola drinks is a potential danger danger during pregnancy.* Some other soft drinks, including Sunkist Orange, Mello Yellow and Mountain Dew, also contain caffeine. Check all soft drink labels for a listing of caffeine. |
| Wine | 1 glass | 90–140 | Traces of some minerals | Potential danger from alcohol.* May act as a diuretic. |
| Beer | 12 oz. | 150 | Carbohydrate<br>Traces of B vitamins | Potential danger from alcohol.* May act as a diuretic. |
| Liquor, martini | 1 glass (3½ oz.) | 140 | None | Potential danger from alcohol.* |

*For an understanding of the potential danger of caffeine and alcohol, see Chapter 8.

group. Pizza, for instance, can be evaluated in terms of its ingredients:

* Crust—grain products
* Cheese—dairy and protein
* Tomato sauce—Vitamin-C–rich vegetable
* Sausage—protein, but also fat

Macaroni and cheese is a combination of dairy, grain and protein. Soups contribute vegetables, protein foods, and dairy items; a raw spinach salad may have spinach (green leafy vegetable), mushrooms (other vegetables), tomatoes (Vitamin-C–rich food), hard-cooked egg (protein), and salad dressing (fats and oils).

With a bit of practice, you will find you can place your food choices into the appropriate categories. Precision is not important; this is just a way to help you get an overall idea of the way your diet balances out. *If a whole group of foods is being regularly neglected, chances are you are missing out on some important nutrients.*

### Surprise Superstars

**LIVER**
☆

Liver is the worst kept nutritional secret. It is the topic of endless jokes. Stop laughing and take another look, because liver appears as a source of almost every important nutrient.

Give it a try; many restaurants have liver and onions or bacon on their menu, if you don't want to prepare it yourself. Liver pâté is an elegant as well as nutritious appetizer. How about a chicken-liver omelet or a liver-sausage sandwich?

The authors of this book like liver thinly sliced and quickly sautéed with peppers, mushrooms, and onions. We celebrate special events at a restaurant that makes liver this way.

If you cannot face it "straight," have the butcher grind a quarter-pound of liver with a pound of ground beef, and cook it as you usually cook ground beef. You won't even know it's there!

**GREENS,** These foods join the proverbial spinach as great
**KALE,** nutritional bargains. All give more than a whole
**BROCCOLI** day's supply of vitamin A, vitamin C, many B vita-
☆ mins, and lots of minerals for less than 50 calories
per serving. Get out your favorite cookbook and
find ways to prepare them!

**CANTA-** Cantaloupe is not only refreshing and delicious,
**LOUPE** but is a good buy when in season. Half of a
☆ medium-size cantaloupe has only 60 calories,
potassium, enough vitamin A and vitamin C for
a whole day, and lots of other vitamins and minerals. Fill a
cantaloupe wedge with cottage cheese, tuna salad, or chicken
salad for a quick and easy meal.

**HEARTY** Hearty soups are good, nutritious convenience
**SOUPS** foods. Split-pea or bean soups, minestrone,
☆ Chunky Turkey and Chunky Vegetable by Camp-
bell's, and similar soups by Heinz and other soup
companies have lots of vegetables giving a variety of nutrients
including Vitamin A and some protein. They only require
heating and are quickly prepared. They have quite a bit of salt,
which should not be a problem during pregnancy. Have some
handy when you do not feel like cooking, and enjoy them with
whole-grain crackers, a wedge of cheese, and a piece of fruit.
The combination is a light but healthful meal that a child or
mate can fix for you. Of course, hearty homemade soups are
great too, if you have the time.

### Mealtimes

Rule #1 for planning your diet during pregnancy is to *eat at
regular times*. This means three main meals a day and two healthful snacks, or five or six smaller meals at regular intervals.

### Breaking the Fast

You may not be a *breakfast* eater—many people are not—but
breakfast is essential during pregnancy. Energy reserves run

low after a long night without food and both you and the baby need refueling. Recent studies suggest that even relatively short fasts—overnight and skipping breakfast, for instance—can make baby hungry even if you are not.

Breakfast does not need to be bacon and eggs or cereal and toast. Your body has no preconceived ideas about what is appropriate for specific meals. If you feel like it, eat a grilled cheese sandwich, cottage cheese and fruit, leftover macaroni and cheese, hot soup, or some tuna salad.

If making breakfast seems like a lot of time and trouble to you, take advantage of quick-to-fix foods like frozen waffles, quick breakfast drinks made with milk, or ready-to-eat muffins and nut breads.

Cereals are an excellent source of vitamins, minerals, and fiber. If you choose a cereal that is not presweetened, you can control the amount of sugar (and calories) you get. Granola-type cereals, thought by many to be very healthful, contain large amounts of sugar and some oil, and are high in calories. A half-cup serving of one popular brand contains 240 calories; a whole cup of cornflakes has only 84 calories. But granola and granola bars are a good food and nutritious snack if you are not having a problem controlling your weight.

The extra few minutes it takes to eat breakfast before you leave in the morning are especially important during pregnancy. On those days when you are running late and must dash off, make it a point to take along a piece of fruit, peanut butter and crackers, a few oatmeal cookies, or a hard-cooked egg to eat on the way.

In many offices, schools, and factories, the midmorning break is a welcome ritual. Consider alternatives to coffee and doughnuts or sweet rolls, if that's been your habit. How about a corn or bran muffin, a piece of fresh fruit, or a glass of milk and a slice of banana-nut bread? The calories may be as high as you would find in the sweet roll, but these foods have higher nutrient density levels and contribute to your overall nutritional needs.

### Lunchtime

Lunch is the meal most frequently eaten away from home. Whether you "brownbag it" or select meals from a cafeteria or

---

### PUTTING LUNCH TO THE TEST

| *A Sample Menu* | *The Nutritional Critique* |
|---|---|
| Ham and cheese sandwich on white bread with mayonnaise and mustard | The sandwich is high in protein, but also high in fat; make adjustments in the amount of fat you eat at other meals this day. Add some lettuce and tomato to the sandwich and order it on whole-grain bread to increase the nutritional value. |
| Potato chips | They won't hurt you, but they won't help you much, either. High in fat, salt, and calories, they contain few nutrients. Better choices of foods to accompany the sandwich are raw vegetables, bean salad, or cole slaw. |
| Brownie | If having a baby means giving up brownies, we'd have a good hedge against population growth! Consider the brownie in light of your total day's intake of fat and calories. At least the nuts have fiber. A brownie for lunch means no rich dessert for dinner. Fresh fruit, on the other hand, is always a good choice for dessert and it is usually available. |
| Cola Drink | How about having your second glass of milk at lunch, or maybe a glass of tomato juice. |

---

restaurant menu, there are choices to be made. Try to evaluate your food selections; even if what you have to choose from does not represent the best of all possible foods, there are always some that are going to be better for you than others.

### The Fast-Food Fetus

In 1980, 35 percent of every food dollar was spent eating away from home. Twenty-five percent of these meals were eaten at fast-food establishments.[4] Though it might cost more than twice as much as you might pay to prepare the same food at home, fast food is a staple in many diets.

Fast-food menus seldom offer a range of foods adequate to meet all of your needs. Without fresh fruits and vegetables, they often lack vitamins A, C, and folacin. Fiber is noticeably absent in highly processed foods. While some may be low in

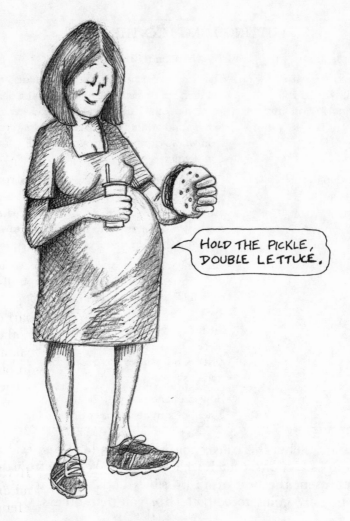

sugar, fast foods are high in both fat and calories. The high
sodium content is a minus for those who should reduce the
total amount of sodium in their diets.

The nutritional pluses may surprise you. Lean ground beef,
chicken, fish, and pizza are good sources of protein; buns, pizza
crusts, and taco shells contribute complex carbohydrates.
Shakes (note, some are not called *milk*shakes) are made of dry
milk solids and contain saturated coconut oil, but they do
supply calcium, riboflavin, niacin, and protein to the diet.

The choices you make from the fast-food menu can tip the

balance of your diet. Here are some guidelines for good choices:

* Eat your burgers without the special sauces that contribute unnecessary fats and calories.
* Add lettuce, tomato, and cheese to your burgers.
* Drink milk instead of a shake, soft drink, tea, or coffee. If milk is not available, the second-best choices are shakes, fruit juice (not fruit drink), lemonade, and water.
* Eat large pieces of fried fish or chicken rather than small ones, which have more batter and retain more fat from frying.
* Accompany your burger with a salad or coleslaw rather than fries when you can.
* Skip the gravy on the mashed potatoes that come with the chicken dinner.
* Go with the original-style chicken; extra crispy is also extra calorie.
* Look at what you eat at a fast-food restaurant as part of the day's total intake and make adjustments at other meals. It may be the day for a bran muffin with breakfast and a large salad at lunch. Try to avoid more than one fried food in the same meal—do not have both fried chicken and fried potatoes.

### Snacking That's Good for You

Snacks are bad for you—right? Well, yes and no. If you snack on foods that contain little more than calories, and are high in sugar, salt, and fat, not much of a nutritional defense can be made for them. However, if your snacks supplement the essential nutrients you need but don't completely get at regular meals, a great deal can be said for them.

Nutritious snacks are ones that are found earlier in this chapter, designated as Best or Other Choices, such as fresh fruit and raw vegetables, banana-nut bread, sunflower seeds, and fruit-flavored yogurt. Some of that milk you are supposed to drink may be enjoyed as a bedtime snack with graham crackers. Popcorn is relatively low in calories (if you skip the butter) and a good source of fiber.

The role of snacks in your diet will depend in large part on your need for calories. Those who need extra calories because of their age or because they were underweight before becoming pregnant may find that they can add to their intake by having several expanded snacks in addition to regular meals. A milkshake, peanut butter and jelly sandwich with a glass of milk, or a dish of cottage cheese with fruit adds both calories and nutrients.

## The "All You Can Eat" Pregnancy Smorgasbord

When you first heard that you were going to need more calories during pregnancy, didn't you think, "Oh, good! Now I don't have to worry about having apple pie for dessert"? The bubble bursts, however, when you find that the added calories are there primarily to ensure adequate intake of essential nutrients.

It is true that in the "perfect diet," 100 percent of the RDAs will be met by choosing prudently from the *Best Choices* food lists; in fact, you will have some calories "left over," and can eat anything you wish.

In the real world, however, most of us do not eat such carefully planned diets, and we do not meet all the RDAs without also consuming plenty of calories. The chances are, *by the time you increase your milk consumption and add an extra vegetable or two that is recommended during pregnancy, you will also have eaten adequate calories.*

## Pregnancy on a Budget

*Eating well during pregnancy is not a luxury, but an investment in your child's future that you cannot afford to neglect.* The Montreal Diet Dispensary mothers improved the outcome of their pregnancies by the mere addition of eggs, milk, and oranges. No additional food costs need be incurred if you are willing to substitute nutritious foods for some of those that contribute little. As you become more aware of the role of eating in relation to health, you will find you are less likely to choose foods merely because you like them, because you are in the habit of buying them, or because you see them advertised.

*Consider your trips to the supermarket as a part of prenatal care.* "I see my doctor once a month; I go to Lamaze classes; I go to the supermarket. . . ." Select foods based on several of the following criteria:

* I like it.
* The rest of my family will eat it.
* It's good for me and the baby.
* It's a good buy this week (check the food pages in the newspaper).
* I know how to prepare the food or have a recipe I'd like to try.
* It's quick and easy.

Then plan your shopping trip.

* Eat before you shop, because everything looks good when you are hungry and you may overspend.
* Select some fresh fruits and vegetables to use right away and others that will keep until the end of the week.
* Do not buy more fresh fruits and vegetables than you can use.
* Prepare a list, but be flexible and try not to make impulse purchases.
* Avoid buying non-nutritious snacks that will only serve as temptation. If all the choices in your refrigerator are good ones, you can't go wrong.
* Purchase some raw fruits and vegetables to keep on hand for munching.
* Get some nonfat dry milk in case you run out of fresh milk.
* Buy milk at the supermarket rather than in smaller, more expensive containers at your neighborhood store.
* Take time to read labels to know what you are getting for your money.
* Try lower-priced brands to see if they will meet your needs.
* Buy some whole-grain crackers and cheese as an alternative to cookies and milk.
* Try at least one new food each week to have a more varied diet.

*Bon Appétit!*

# 8.
# Playing It Safe

The answers are in the chapter and on page 233.

## QUICK QUIZ

The answers are in the chapter and on page 233.

**True or False**

——————  1. Herbal tea is a good alternative to drinking coffee during pregnancy.

——————  2. Switching to low tar/nicotine cigarettes eliminates all risk to the fetus.

——————  3. The *rate* at which you drink alcohol influences the level of risk to your baby.

——————  4. Most diet colas contain caffeine.

——————  5. Birth defects from alcohol occur only if a woman consumes ten drinks or more a day.

——————  6. Babies born to mothers who drink heavily during pregnancy may be smaller at birth, but they soon catch up if they are well fed.

——————  7. The fetus is most likely to be harmed by medication during the first three months of pregnancy.

——————  8. Smoking is more dangerous to your baby in the second half of pregnancy than in the first.

——————  9. Tonic and club soda are both high in caffeine.

—————— 10. Marijuana has recently been proved safe for use by pregnant women.

The time to be concerned about your child's exposure to alcohol, smoking, and drugs cannot be put off until he is a teenager; the time is *now*, if you are pregnant—or are considering having a baby.

It was once thought that the placenta completely protected the fetus from harmful substances. Now we know that many elements, including some that are potentially toxic, can readily pass through the placenta to the baby. If you are concerned about what a beer will do to a teenager, consider what it might do to a fetus! The alcohol in that glass of wine you drink or the caffeine in that cup of coffee can reach your unborn baby within minutes.

## Caffeine: A Stimulating Issue During Pregnancy

Almost everyone in the United States consumes some form of caffeine every day. If you drink caffeine-containing beverages or eat foods containing caffeine when you are pregnant, your baby will be exposed to this chemical even before he is born. This sounds dangerous—is it?

The Surgeon General of the U.S. and the FDA advises mothers-to-be to use caffeine products sparingly.[102] The problem is that there is no way of knowing how much is too much. Total abstinence during pregnancy is not justified, argues the American Council on Science and Health (an association of scientists who evaluate chemicals, the environment, and public health); "moderation" is their recommendation. They emphasize that there is no evidence linking caffeine to birth defects in humans.[150]

Dr. Stephanie Crocco, a food scientist in the Food and Nutrition Department of the American Medical Association, cautions, "An individual's sensitivity to caffeine can vary greatly, making it difficult to recommend general levels of consumption. Additionally, people sometimes forget that cup and mug sizes vary."

What's a mother to do?

There are several questions to consider that will help you decide on a course of action: What do we know about the

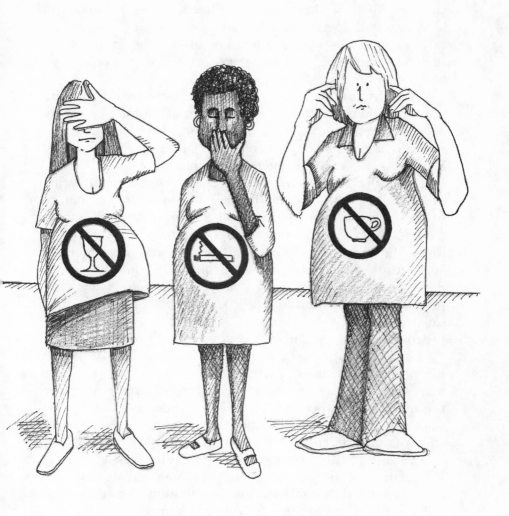

effects of caffeine during pregnancy? How much caffeine do *you* consume?

More than forty animal studies with caffeine have been conducted in the past thirty to forty years. Large quantities of the chemical (equivalent to twenty to a hundred cups of coffee a day) have produced birth defects in rats, mice, rabbits, and chickens. Because these negative effects can be produced in several animal species, and because the seriousness of defects can be correlated with the amount of caffeine given, many researchers feel there is ample reason to send up the yellow flag of warning for pregnant women.[150]

The Institute of Nutrition at the University of North Carolina points out that: "Consumption of caffeine has yet to be established as toxic to human fetuses. However, any substance that crosses the placenta may be regarded as possibly hazardous, especially during the first trimester. . . ."[151B]

Does caffeine affect human babies as it affects the offspring in animal studies? During the past ten years, a number of studies have attempted to show this. However, because human mothers cannot be treated like mice or rabbits, it is difficult to isolate the effects of caffeine. Many women who consume large amounts of caffeine also smoke, drink alcohol, and have poor diets. Some of these women have miscarriages, stillbirths, premature births, and babies born with birth defects. The caffeine may have contributed to the poor outcome of their pregnancies, but we cannot say it caused the problems.

There is an additional problem facing the scientists on this matter of caffeine in pregnancy. To be sure that the risks they may warn about are real risks, scientists studying the chemicals use animals that process the chemical in a manner similar to the way humans process the same chemical. In other words, scientists use the chemically appropriate animal model. Currently, scientists are not sure how to interpret their laboratory information about caffeine because each animal studied processes caffeine differently and all of these study animals process caffeine somewhat differently from the human.

We do know, however, that caffeine passes quickly into the human bloodstream, ready to stimulate your tired brain and muscles—and your baby. The caffeine you drink when you are pregnant can pass into the circulatory system of the baby.[151B] It tends to build up to a more concentrated level in the baby because the fetus cannot process it as efficiently as the mother's system does.[150] Unlike alcohol, which dehydrates cells, caffeine stimulates cells. Many scientists believe that more research is needed to determine the risks.

In addition, there are side effects of caffeine-containing beverages that make large quantities undesirable during pregnancy. Many of these foods, such as coffee and tea, contain acids that can irritate the digestive tract. In addition, caffeine stimulates the secretion of acid in the stomach. This does not spell R-E-L-I-E-F, but indigestion and heartburn.

Kidneys produce more urine when high levels of caffeine are present, which results in the loss of fluids, vitamins, and minerals that are needed by both mother and baby during pregnancy.

### What Will It Be, Madame—Coffee, Tea, Cola, or Excedrin?

Most of us consume a lot more caffeine than we think we do.

As we write this chapter, burning the late-night oil, we suddenly realize that the mug on the desk contains a good bit more than the 5-ounce portion in a traditional coffee cup. A trip to the kitchen to take a measurement reveals that our "cup" of coffee is, in fact, *10 ounces* of coffee! How many of these "cups" do we say we drink in a day (or night)? Actually, many of us would be hard-pressed to say, perhaps because we add a little to the cup to "warm it up" every time we pass the pot. Those of us who have access to a continual supply are most likely to get hooked by this habit.

If you are feeling smug because you drink *tea*, you are in for a surprise. While many teas contain less caffeine than coffee, there are some that contain more than coffee. The tea connoisseur who likes loose, imported tea in a full-strength brew is the one most likely to be on the heavy end of that scale. The "bag-in-bag-out" drinker gets considerably less caffeine in her cup. Tea also contains *theophylline*, a close chemical relative of caffeine.

Recent concerns about caffeine have led to the development of *decaffeinated coffees*. "Decaf" may take a little getting used to, but taste tests have shown that there are a number of acceptable products, especially when the decafs are of the brewed rather than the instant types. These decaffeinated products do reduce the amount of caffeine to virtually nothing, but some of the acids that cause indigestion and heartburn remain.

If you are a coffee or tea drinker, try decaffeinated brands during pregnancy as a way of limiting your caffeine consumption. Caffeine is not "addictive" in the same way nicotine is, but if you abruptly cut back on consumption, you may experience unpleasant symptoms such as headache, nervousness, or irritability.[150] One way to avoid these reactions is to mix the decaffeinated tea or coffee with your regular brand, gradually increasing the proportion of the decaffeinated product until you have adjusted to the new taste and level of stimulation. It may make it a little harder to "get going" in the morning, but you will probably sleep better at night!

Some women may be concerned about potential hazards resulting from the use of chemicals in decaffeinating. Most manufacturers in this country use methylene chloride to extract the caffeine. An analysis by Consumers Union showed that no residues remained in the finished product.[4]

*Herbal teas*, seen as an alternative to caffeine-containing tea by a growing number in this country, may not be the sweet, innocent health drink they purport to be. Many contain substances that can cause vomiting, diarrhea, heart palpitations, lowered blood pressure, and allergic reactions. While some herbal teas may be safe, if drunk occasionally, prolonged use may be a hazard to health.[4] Some herbal teas contain known toxins, but they are not likely to be banned by the Food and Drug Administration because these substances are naturally occurring as opposed to being added during processing. Scientists warn not to use herbal teas that lack adequate information about ingredients on the label and not to drink large amounts of herbal teas in strongly brewed solutions. While there is no research specifically related to the effect of herbal teas on the fetus, herbal teas should be considered as druglike, and drugs should always be viewed as questionable during pregnancy.

The caffeine removed from decaffeinated coffee beans does not necessarily go to "waste." Some may be sold to the soft drink industry, and recycled into *soft drinks*. Until recently, the FDA Standards of Identity required that when beverages called themselves "colas" or "pepper" drinks, they had to contain caffeine. The FDA is now in the process of changing this regulation, and several companies are developing caffeine-free colas. Most ginger ales and some fruit-flavored drinks do not contain caffeine. Check the labels on all soft drinks for caffeine content.

In 1975, cola beverages accounted for 64 percent of regular soft drink sales, and per-capita consumption of soft drinks was calculated at 3,512 ounces, about triple the intake of 1955. [39] When you think that this is per-capita consumption (the amount sold in the United States, divided by the total number of men, women, and children) and that many people never drink soft drinks, the amount of soft drinks consumed by those who drink significant quantities is staggering.

Diet soft drink users may think they do not need to be concerned about caffeine. On the contrary; the saccharin in diet soft drinks is a substitute for sugar, not caffeine. In fact, there are more reasons to avoid diet drinks than regular soft drinks during pregnancy. Saccharin has yet to be declared risk-free for humans; its major use is for diabetics and to control weight gain, and during pregnancy you want to gain some weight! We do not yet know whether artificial sweeteners have effects on future generations of humans. Why should you let yourself be a guinea pig?

Though we cannot blame caffeine for the "addiction" some people seem to have for chocolate, there are significant amounts in chocolate products. Chocolate's "active ingredient" is *theobromine*, a substance that has physiologic actions and a chemical structure similar to caffeine, but its action on the nervous system is slightly different. A typical cup of cocoa contains less than 20 milligrams of caffeine, but over 200 milligrams of theobromine. That hot cocoa you drink just before bed to help you sleep may in fact have just the opposite effect!

Over-the-counter drugs can be another major source of caffeine in the typical American diet. "But," you say, "drugs don't count as part of the diet." Anything that goes into your mouth and through your digestive system is "diet." Whether caffeine is coming from a cup of coffee or an aspirin-type product makes little difference to the way the caffeine is processed by your body and the effect it can have on your baby is the same.

Examine the chart that shows amounts of caffeine in foods and drugs to determine how much caffeine you consume. If the amount is high enough to warrant altering your habits, try the suggestions on page 157.

| CAFFEINE COUNTER [34] | | |
|---|---|---|
| Food | Portion | Milligrams Caffeine |
| **Coffee:** Brewed | 8 oz. | 85–200 |
| Percolated | 8 oz. | 97–125 |
| Drip | 8 oz. | 137–153 |
| Instant (Mellow Roast, Nescafé, Taster's Choice, Yuban) | 8 oz. | 50–60 |
| Decaffeinated (Brim, Taster's Choice, Sanka) | 8 oz. | 3–5 |
| Freeze-dried (Maxim) | 1 tsp. | 61 |
| Café Francais, Vienna, Suisse Mocha | 1 tsp. | 29–32 |
| **Cocoa:** Hot chocolate | 8 oz. | 6–42 |
| Cocoa, dry | 1 Tbsp. | 9–14 |
| **Tea:** (each brewed 5 minutes): | | |
| Green | 8 oz. | 31–35 |
| Oolong | 8 oz. | 24–40 |
| Instant | 8 oz. | 30 |
| Constant Comment | 8 oz. | 31 |
| Caffeine-Free (Boston's) | 8 oz. | 9 |
| Earl Gray | 8 oz. | 61 |
| Regular (Grand Union, Harvest Day, Pantry Pride, Royal Jewel) | 8 oz. | 40–50 |
| Regular (Red Rose, Canterbury, Lipton, Our-Own, Salada, Stewarts, White Rose) | 8 oz. | 50–60 |
| Regular (Tender Leaf, Tetley, Twinings) | 8 oz. | 60–66 |
| **Soft Drinks:** Cola, Coca Cola | 12 oz. | 30–90 |
| Diet Rite | 12 oz. | 33 |
| Dr. Pepper, regular and sugar-free | 12 oz. | 54–61 |
| Mountain Dew, Mr. Pibb | 12 oz. | 55–57 |
| Pepsi Cola, Pepsi Light | 12 oz. | 36 |
| Royal Crown | 12 oz. | 21–34 |
| RC-100 | 12 oz. | 0 |
| Tab | 12 oz. | 45 |
| **Drugs:** Dristan, Sinarest, Aspirin with caffeine Cope, Midol | | 30–32/pill |
| Excedrin, Anacin, Pre-Mens | | 60–66/pill |
| No Doz, Vivarin | | 100–200/pill |

To limit caffeine:
* *Count* the cups or mugs of coffee or tea you drink to avoid casual overconsumption.
* *Choose* beverages that contain *no* caffeine (fruit juices, vegetable juices, milk, tonic, club soda, water).
* *Reduce* the amount of caffeine by drinking decaffeinated coffee or tea.
* *Change* the method by which you prepare coffee; brew tea for a short period of time.
* *Drink* noncaffeinated soft drinks, if you must drink them at all.
* *Avoid* taking medications, if at all possible, and take only those your doctor prescribes or permits.

Both of us drank coffee during our pregnancies. It was a nice, sociable, low-calorie beverage for Anne at home, and Mary at work. Since neither of us likes soft drinks, the general choice of daily beverages was juice, milk, and coffee. Anne drank some water, too; Mary drank hot or iced tea. Neither of us can identify any problem associated with the coffee we consumed. Both of us still drink significant quantities of coffee and tea. How real is the risk to you? To us? We are just not sure.

How much caffeine is too much is a very individual matter. Dr. Keith Russell, Clinical Professor of Obstetrics and Gynecology at the University of California, and a past president of the American College of Obstetricians and Gynecologists, tells his patients to pare coffee consumption to a maximum of one to two cups a day.[139] The Food and Drug Administration suggests that adults (not pregnant women) limit caffeine to 400 milligrams a day, or about six cups of coffee.[139] The FDA has not set a safety limit for pregnant women.

## Food Additives—An Added Hazard?

Food additives and fetuses just don't sound as though they belong in the same womb. Most of us have learned to accept a little sodium propionate in our bread and a judicious bit of propylene glycol monostearate in our salad dressing, but what happens to an unborn child if it gets a dose of an antimicrobial additive or emulsifier?

The Food and Drug Administration requires that any new substance be subjected to tests designed to simulate situations that could produce ill-effects. The problem is that these tests must be conducted with animals, and there is always a remote possibility of humans' reacting differently, or of an individual's having a lower level of tolerance. Some substances have been used for many years but have never been thoroughly tested—salt, BHT, and BHA, for instance. Some are undergoing further tests; others have been declared safe on the basis of current scientific knowledge. *There are no cases that document that commonly used food additives are dangerous during pregnancy.*

The scientific data that have been accumulated so far do not support strict avoidance of specific food additives. Nevertheless, there is the public perception that food additives should be avoided during pregnancy. Of particular concern to consumers are nitrites, artificial colors and flavors, monosodium glutamate, and artificial sweeteners. Let's look at these.

*Nitrites* are added to cured meats. Nitrites are converted to Nitrosamines when bacon is fried at very high temperatures. *Nitrosamines* are a potential carcinogen and consuming them is a realistic concern. Whether there is specific risk to the unborn child has not been determined, but since bacon is not on the "Best Choice" lists of foods for pregnancy, you can easily avoid it or limit consumption.

*Artificial colors and flavors* have been extensively studied. These substances have not been correlated with any birth defects or complications of pregnancy.

*Monosodium glutamate* (MSG) is a chemical used as a flavor enhancer. Many people use "Accent," which is a product name for MSG. MSG is frequently used in Chinese and Japanese cooking. The concern about MSG was raised because some mice fed huge amounts of MSG developed brain lesions. There is no evidence that MSG, as normally consumed, crosses the placenta or is transmitted in breast milk.[167]

*Saccharin, cyclamates*, and *aspartame* are all artificial sweeteners. Saccharin is used in low-calorie and dietetic products in the

United States. The law requires that whenever it is used, it must be clearly labeled. Cyclamate is used in Canada. Aspartame is a new non-nutritive sweetener derived from protein. It has recent-been approved for sale in the United States and has passed all of the tests except the effects of long-term use by humans.

When saccharin was tested for safety, it was found that after several generations of high saccharin intake, a few rats developed cancer of the bladder. Again, we do not know what this means to humans. Since artificial sweeteners are fairly easy to avoid, it seems reasonable to omit the foods that contain them. This may turn out to be an unnecessary restriction as more data become available, but you cannot wait ten years for an answer to the question of safety during your pregnancy.

The whole area of food additives in pregnancy is one where there seem to be a lot of suspicions but few facts and conclusions. If you follow the suggestions in the Nutrition Game Plan, and select from the *Best Choices* lists, your diet will be relatively low in food additives. *A good rule of thumb is to use as many fresh, whole foods as possible and generally to limit the fabricated, high-technology alternatives.* There is very little room in your diet for the highly sugared, caloried, or fried snack items that are loaded with additives.

## Warning:
## Cigarette Smoke Is Dangerous to Your Unborn Baby's Health

The Surgeon General's Advisory warning to smokers appears on every pack of cigarettes, though few smokers are deterred by it. During pregnancy, the warning must be extended to include the baby, who smokes when you do. Do you really want your baby to smoke?

A recent national survey of college students revealed that 31 percent of females and 21 percent of males were cigarette smokers.[115] If you smoke, you certainly have plenty of company.

Research shows that smoking is a significant risk to completing pregnancy and delivering a healthy child. The effects of smoking are listed on the next page.

Maternal smoking during pregnancy:

* raises the amount of energy you expend, which increases the need for calories. Smoking accelerates heartbeat and oxygen need.[172A]
* increases the likelihood of spontaneous abortion and miscarriage.[81]
* results in 50 percent more premature deliveries than in nonsmoking mothers and more than twice as many low-birth-weight babies.[2]
* doubles a woman's risk of aborting or having a stillborn baby.[164]
* may have long-term effects on the child's mental and physical well-being.[17]

Early work suggests that 20 percent of babies who died prior to or within a few weeks after delivery might have lived if the mother had not smoked during pregnancy.[112] Infants born of parents who smoke have double the incidence of bronchitis and pneumonia in the first year of life.[168]

*How much you smoke does make a difference.* Studies show that the birth weight of babies is proportional to the number of cigarettes smoked,[110] though even light smoking (four or five cigarettes a day) results in babies that weigh less than those of non-smoking mothers.[2] There is some evidence that mothers who stop smoking or significantly reduce their smoking by the fifth month of pregnancy spare their babies possible damage.[153]

One of the major reasons why smoking is discouraged during pregnancy is that it suppresses the appetite. The two thousand chemicals in cigarette smoke may satisfy your hunger, but they don't provide the essential nutrients that are necessary to produce a healthy baby!

### Nicotine, Tar, and Carbon Monoxide

The nicotine in cigarettes speeds up your heartbeat by ten to twenty beats a minute, and smoking even one cigarette can produce a sudden speeding-up, then slowing-down of the fetal heartbeat.[2]

Nicotine causes arteries to contract, so blood flows more slowly and laboriously through the constricted channels, making you feel tired and weak. Nicotine makes the arteries in the wall of the uterus contract, reducing the flow of blood to the placenta. If this happens, some of the cells in the uterus may die and the attachment between the placenta and the uterus can weaken.

Many smokers have switched to low-tar/nicotine cigarettes, which is probably a good thing, but not good enough for pregnancy.[164] Generally people build up a nicotine tolerance level, and many may smoke more of the low-tar/nicotine cigarettes than regular ones that have higher nicotine and tar values.

A major hazard of smoking is carbon monoxide, which is not reduced in low-tar/nicotine cigarettes. It is a poison that slows down the flow of oxygen in your blood, therefore reducing the oxygen supply to the fetus. Ultrasonic monitoring has shown reduced fetal movement after the mother smoked two cigarettes successively.

The Public Health Service of the United States in its report "Health Consequences of Smoking, 1975," after recounting statistics that indicate that smokers have smaller babies, said: "These effects may occur because carbon monoxide passes freely across the placenta and is readily bound by fetal hemoglobin, thereby decreasing the oxygen-carrying capacity of fetal blood."[164]

### The Smoke-Filled Womb

Research shows that if you do not smoke, but are continually breathing in secondhand smoke, your heartbeat increases and your blood pressure goes up. For this reason, you should even avoid smoke-filled rooms when you are pregnant. There is pressure on people these days to stop smoking, so you probably will not meet with resistance if you tell someone nicely that the smoke bothers you, and ask that he or she please put out the cigarette.

If you are timid, you might try doing what our friend Jeanne Helmrick does. She tells annoying smokers that the smoke is making her nauseated. If you add that you are pregnant, they will be quick to comply with your request!

*If you are having a baby, both you and your mate will want to protect the health of your baby by providing a smoke-free environment. If you can't quit, at least cut down on your smoking. Make your motto "A cleaner world; a healthier family."*

## To Drink or Not to Drink?

This is *not* a new problem. Ancient Spartans forbade young married couples from drinking because they found it produced less than healthy babies. The Bible warns pregnant women not to drink alcohol.[24] Thus, history shows that pregnancy has carried with it restrictions about alcohol consumption. Because drinking is important in our social lives, many of us have chosen to ignore the warnings. On behalf of your baby, however, we present the following information.

Your body does not react to ethyl alcohol like any other substance you eat or drink. First, ethyl alcohol (the alcohol found in beer, wines, and distilled liquor) is absorbed more quickly than any of the nutrients. It is rapidly transported to the liver, where it is processed and changed into energy at the rate of 7 calories per gram (compare that to 4 calories per gram in carbohydrate or protein and 9 calories per gram in fats). These calories are limited in their usefulness, however. No cells, except those in the liver, can process the potential calories in ethyl alcohol.[46]

The liver can handle only limited amounts of ethyl alcohol at a time. It can completely process only about a third of an ounce of alcohol an hour;[46] that's an hour and a half to two hours to metabolize the alcohol in one 12-ounce can of beer! If you eat as you drink, and sip your drink over a period of time, you may be able to slow down the rate of absorption and keep alcohol at levels that can be processed by the liver. If an "overload" occurs, the excess alcohol circulates in the bloodstream until the liver can handle it. Some is excreted; some evaporates as it passes through the lung (and can be smelled on a person's breath). While in the bloodstream, it affects every organ it passes. It goes through the placenta and into the circulatory system of the fetus.[39]

### Alcohol and the Unborn Child

Your body doesn't know whether the alcohol you drink comes from a martini, a beer, a glass of wine, or a cold remedy. Many mouthwashes, cough syrups, cold remedies, and liquid pain relievers contain substantial amounts of alcohol. Ask your doctor to suggest products safe for you to use. If children's preparations are suggested, it is because most of them are formulated without alcohol. *Read the labels!*

---

### EQUIVALENT AMOUNTS OF ALCOHOL
#### (About 0.5 ounce pure alcohol) [165]

*1 drink =*

| | |
|---|---|
| 1 jigger, 1½ oz. | Liquor: whiskey, rum, gin, vodka, scotch, etc. |
| 1 glass, 5 oz. | Wine: dry table wine, red or white |
| 10-oz. glass | Beer |
| 12-oz glass | Beer: light types |

---

Nobody can predict what damage may occur if a woman drinks only once in a while or has an occasional evening of heavier drinking. The evidence on the effects of moderate or occasional drinking is unclear. We do not know a safe level for drinking at this time. Jennie Kline at Columbia University said, "Neither the birth-weight finding nor the spontaneous abortion finding is so secure that women should feel guilty if they take a drink. As scientists, I don't think any of us believe that a little bit of alcohol causes these effects."[100A]

Many physicians, with years of experience with pregnant women who have had an occasional drink and had no problems, are not particularly concerned if a well-nourished pregnant woman has a drink once in a while.[172A] The problem is excess. Whenever you drink to excess, you may be exposing your baby to danger.

We all know women who have had wine or a drink many evenings of their pregnancy and have had perfectly normal, healthy children. In the years when we were pregnant, the risks of alcohol abuse during pregnancy were not documented as they are now; and both of us had an occasional glass of wine without even a pang of conscience. Our babies were just fine, too. In retrospect it seems ironic that, in those days, it was usual to serve wine or alcoholic punch at baby showers!

The American Council on Science and Health has recently reviewed the scientific literature about alcohol usage during pregnancy. Their report states,

"Studies have found no increase in the frequency of physical abnormalities at levels up to one ounce of absolute alcohol, or an average of two drinks, daily. No study can prove an absolute safe level of drinking. But for this consumption level, the risks, if any, appear to be low.[150A]

They go on to explain that a woman should limit her consumption to this level and particularly avoid binge drinking. The relationship between birth defects and alcohol becomes uncertain as levels of alcohol increase. Drinking levels between one and five ounces of pure alcohol daily have shown increased risk of low birth weights, miscarriages, and lowered intelligence scores. But there is no consistent pattern of extent or pattern of damage. Also the risk of drinking is greatly increased if the mother also smokes cigarettes.[150A]

When five or more ounces of alcohol, about 10 drinks, are consumed daily, there is a possibility of fetal alcohol syndrome. The term *fetal alcohol syndrome* (FAS), was first used in 1973 to describe a recognizable pattern of physical and mental birth defects in many babies born to women who are chronic alcoholics. It is estimated that at least 8 percent of American women of childbearing age are alcoholics.[100A] *Babies with true FAS are born to women who are chronic alcoholics, not to well-nourished women who have an occasional glass of wine!*

Babies with FAS are abnormally small at birth, especially in head size, and they do not have the same amount of brain tissue as normal children.[132] If alcohol prevents cell-division and growth, the brain simply does not develop to fill out the head. The eyes are too close together and are covered by a fold of skin at the inner corners; there is virtually no bridge to the nose; and the space above the lip is flat. The affected children are severely mentally retarded and usually have emotional problems; about half have heart defects.[165]

Many of these babies are irritable and jittery in the first few days after birth as they begin their lives with alcohol withdrawal. As they grow, they have behavioral problems and short attention spans, and are poorly coordinated.[92] They fail to gain adequate weight, even if given a nutritious diet. They never catch up.

Not every baby with FAS has all of the defects, and not every woman who drinks heavily gives birth to a baby with FAS. There are also more subtle effects of alcohol consumption, which may not result in full FAS but can cause mild to moderate mental and physical retardation, inability to concentrate, hyperactivity, and behavioral or sleep problems that are not apparent until the child grows older.[160] This is called *fetal alcohol effects* or *modified FAS*.

About 30 to 50 percent of chronic alcoholic mothers deliver babies with FAS, making it the third-ranking known cause of birth defects and one that leads to mental retardation. *Unlike most other birth defects, FAS is preventable.* The March of Dimes Birth Defects Foundation has been doing excellent work in providing guidance to prevent birth defects. Their local chapter and publications can be a valuable resource to you.

In July of 1981, the Surgeon General's Advisory included a warning: *Women who are pregnant or even considering pregnancy should avoid alcohol completely and should be aware of the alcoholic content of food and drugs.*[76] The "even considering pregnancy" is added because many women do not know they are pregnant in the first few weeks, which is a period of rapid cell division and a time of high vulnerability. Physicians were told to warn their patients. The alcoholic beverage industry has been advised to make the risks known.

The conservative approach of the Surgeon General's Advisory grows out of studies demonstrating that, while women who have five or more drinks a day (see table) are most at risk, even moderate drinking is associated with retarded fetal growth.[165] Individual women may process alcohol more or less efficiently, and some fetuses may be more or less susceptible to the toxic effects of alcohol. If the fetus happens to be at a critical stage of development, your drinking can be harmful. The Surgeon General advised that sizable and significant increases in spontaneous abortions have been observed in pregnant women who drank as little as 2 ounces of alcohol twice a week.[132] *The truth is that no one knows how little or how much alcohol can damage an unborn baby.*

### Nutrient Robber Barons

In addition to the potential dangers posed by drinking, it can jeopardize the supply of essential nutrients needed for baby-building. Vitamins (especially thiamin and niacin) are used to process alcohol in the liver. This alcohol-processing use prevents these same vitamins from being used to convert glucose into energy or protein into tissues. In addition, drinking often causes increased excretion and urination, which can flush vitamins, minerals, and fluids out of the mother's body, denying them to both mother and baby. Heavy drinkers tend to be deficient in two very important nutrients for pregnancy— iron and folic acid.

One of the greatest dangers of alcohol is that alcohol substitutes just calories for foods and nutrients in your diet. A nourishing meal may be replaced by a munchy snack or another drink.

Do you still want a drink?

When Anne's friend Susan was pregnant, she used to tell her friends at parties, "No, thank you. Today is the day my baby's IQ is going from 120 to 130."

## Drugs—Taking Them and Doing Them

One definition of a *drug* is that it is a chemical that helps with the diagnosis, cure, prevention, or treatment of an illness. But what is given to heal sometimes proves to be a hazard. Women who took thalidomide, an apparently harmless tranquilizer used as a sleeping pill, produced horribly malformed babies. Another frightening discovery was made when it was learned that the daughters of women who took a hormone called DES, to prevent miscarrying, were found to have a much greater incidence of cancer of the vagina and cervix. The Food and Drug Administration (FDA) requires extensive testing of potential hazards of drugs; many drugs contain warnings on the labels against use during pregnancy. Physicians avoid prescribing medications during pregnancy, if at all possible, especially during the first three months. However, you should not be afraid to take medications if they are needed and prescribed by your doctor; both you and the baby must be kept healthy.

*Do not take any medication without consulting your doctor or nurse.* The doctor has lists of medications that have been proved safe or unsafe in pregnancy and lactation,[45,142] *but you must ask!*

Even "everyday" over-the-counter drugs must be carefully screened for use during pregnancy. The innocent cold tablet or aspirin can have a negative effect.

Over 20 billion *aspirin* tablets are consumed yearly in this country, making aspirin America's most widely used drug.[136] A study of over fifty thousand pregnant women found that 64 percent of them used aspirin during their pregnancy.[62] The salicylate in aspirin crosses the placenta freely, and can be found in the fetal bloodstream at birth.

Research indicates that aspirin may interfere with the development of normal circulation in the fetus and newborn,[131] increase the risk of hemorrhage to the mother and newborn,[136] and delay the onset of labor and extend its duration.[136]

The Food and Drug Administration's Advisory Panel on Over-the-Counter Analgesics has recommended that women be warned not to take aspirin during the last three months of pregnancy unless under the advice and supervision of a physician.[136]

Women who have a condition requiring constant medication are advised to discuss the implications with their doctor or a specialist *prior to* becoming pregnant. If you take *birth control pills*, it is best to stop using them at least three months before you attempt to conceive. If you become pregnant—or even think you are pregnant—while taking "The Pill," stop immediately, and consult your doctor.

*Barbiturates* such as *Nembutal,* and *Seconal* (yellow jackets, nemmies, yellows, reds, seccy, red devils) and tranquilizers, such as *Valium, Librium, Tranxene,* and *Serax,* cross the placenta, thereby presenting a risk to the fetus.[22] Both barbiturates and tranquilizers can create a *fetal* dependency on the drug, and drug-dependent newborns suffer withdrawal symptoms. Although the short-term effects can be controlled by medication, there is no research showing the possible long-range effects. An association between Valium and cleft-palate has been reported when the drug was used during the first trimester of pregnancy.[22] This is especially noteworthy because the beginning weeks of pregnancy are often stressful as hormonal balances shift and moods change readily. If you take barbiturates or tranquilizers, give them up before you become pregnant. If you are already pregnant, seek the advice of someone who can help you stop.

Though most people do not think of them as such, nicotine and alcohol are often considered drugs. A number of women have given up or reduced their use of nicotine and alcohol in favor of other social drugs such as marijuana.

*Marijuana* is the most widely used "soft" drug in the United States. Marijuana is rapidly absorbed from the lungs into the bloodstream, where it is then processed by many tissues (unlike alcohol, which is processed only by the liver). Unfortunately, the active ingredients are stored in fat deposits and are excreted over a period of time. It takes a week or more after smoking even one joint for the residue to completely clear the body.

Women tend not to mention their use of marijuana to their physicians, so it is generally not even considered as a possible cause of a particular problem. There is concern about the effects of marijuana use on chromosomes—some research and clinical reports find abnormalities, while others do not. It has been speculated that regular use of marijuana by a pregnant woman may have specific effects on the potential hormonal levels of a male fetus.[93]

There is no conclusive evidence to date that marijuana is harmful to the fetus or causes problems in labor or delivery.[22] We hasten to point out that because marijuana is not legal, the content of marijuana preparations is not subject to standards or control of the FDA. Some marijuana may contain considerably more THC, the hallucinogenic agent, than others. It may be contaminated with pesticides or contain "hard drugs." Visual examination cannot detect this.

You may be one of the growing number who are using *cocaine*. Cocaine, along with nicotine and amphetamines, is a stimulant. Though no research has shown the risks of cocaine to the fetus, the dangers of nicotine are well established, and amphetamines may have the potential to cause birth defects.[111] So why take a chance by using any of these stimulants?

In doing research for this book, we asked doctors and nutritionists many questions. We asked two prominent researchers about the potential effects of cocaine on fetal development. There were no specific answers to be found. Why? Because most women do not tell their doctors that they use cocaine or other illegal drugs. There are no controlled study populations, and there is little information in medical journals. This does not mean that there are not significant negative effects—women were having "Fetal Alcohol Syndrome" babies for years but we did not identify the problem until 1973, despite the fact that it is both obvious and serious.

*Hard drugs,* such as cocaine, heroin, morphine, and PCP, invite more problems than pleasure during pregnancy. Money that should be spent for food may be diverted to buy drugs. The behavior of a mother-to-be who uses drugs may result in harm to her and her baby—and there are the unknown risks to the unborn child.

The conclusion that Oakley Ray, professor of psychology at Vanderbilt University, reaches is, "There must be the warning that it is unwise for a pregnant woman to use any non-essential drug at any level because of the possibility of effects on the fetus."[39]

*There are situations during pregnancy that warrant taking a drug—but only when it benefits the mother or the unborn child, and only under a physician's supervision.* Casual or social use of medicinal or narcotic substances cannot be justified.

Each of us is responsible for her choices in food, drugs, and most every action in life. During pregnancy, you are also responsible for the choices you make on behalf of your baby. This is a time for caution. A short-term commitment during pregnancy can minimize the chances of your baby being born with birth defects or health problems that may limit his potential and create a lifetime of problems. It isn't always easy, but it can be done. Cathy, a recent first-time mother, recalls her experience. "When I became pregnant, I developed terrible cravings for certain things I knew I should not have. By the end of pregnancy, I had a *mad desire* to drink a whole pot of strong coffee, eat a pound of chocolate and get drunk!"

When asked if she did any of these things, she replied, "I did allow myself one cup of coffee each morning when I was pregnant, but I gave up alcohol completely. The minute I delivered, my cravings disappeared." Ryan Benjamin is a wonderful, healthy baby. He is the most brilliant and beautiful of all the grandchildren, his Grandma Abbott proclaimed. But then, Grandma Abbott says that about each of her grand-children.

# 9.
# Special
# Needs of
# Pregnancy

There is nothing very beautiful or fulfilling about morning sickness—or hemorrhoids, constipation, or swollen ankles, for that matter. Considering all the changes that take place in your body during pregnancy, it is no wonder that some women experience discomforts and occasional complications. If you understand why a particular physical reaction occurs, and know what to do about it, at least you will not be frightened if it happens to you.

*In this chapter, we will discuss the problems in pregnancy that are specifically related to your diet.*

## The Ups and Downs of Pregnancy

### Nausea/Vomiting

"I was one of those women who believed that morning sickness was all psychological," Anne recalls. "That was because it never happened to me! Then I spent a day with a newly

171

pregnant friend who was experiencing her sixth consecutive day of vomiting. I knew then that it was not 'all in the head!' "
There are some instances when morning sickness is psychosomatic, but for the two out of three pregnant women who have morning sickness, it is physically very real.

*Mary*: "I had been told that I could not have children. While traveling in Europe, I got a 'flu' that made me sick, tired, and irritable, especially in the morning. I thought it was related to the water and not sleeping well at night. A friend suggested that I have my urine tested because she was *sure* I was pregnant. When the test came back positive, I don't know who was more shocked—Peter, my doctor or I!

"So I know that it isn't psychosomatic—my body sent me a message that I didn't hear. But it also helps me to understand how some women know that they are pregnant in the first few weeks. I guess when you consider pregnancy a possibility, you get the message more quickly."

The not-so-wonderful thing about morning sickness is that, although it usually occurs in the morning, you can experience it any time of the day or night—or, on occasion, for a whole day or night. It is usually over at about the twelfth week of pregnancy, but don't be surprised if you are nauseated on day #100.

*Cause*: Scientists do not know for sure what causes nausea and vomiting in early pregnancy, but changing hormone levels are thought to contribute to the condition. HCG, the hormone that indicates pregnancy in urine tests, is at high levels during the first trimester. As it decreases, nausea also decreases, which may indicate a cause-and-effect relationship.[73]

Low levels of maternal blood sugar, which signal "time to eat," ironically combine with a slowing down of the digestive process. This is Nature's way of increasing the efficiency of nutrient intake during pregnancy. Eating foods slowly seems to help. Some women experience great anxiety and stress when they find they are pregnant, which can interfere with their digestion of foods. Nausea has also been attributed to low levels of B vitamins, especially $B_6$ and thiamin.[107]

While nausea is not pleasant, the real danger in vomiting is that the combination of reduced food intake and a loss of fluids can lead to weakness and dehydration. Often nausea can be controlled so that vomiting does not occur.

The traditional advice to nauseated pregnant women is to eat crackers. Beatrice Briggs remembers, "I've never eaten so many crackers in my life as I did during my first three months of pregnancy! I still feel nauseated when I see a box of saltines."

*What to Do If You are Nauseated*
* Eat frequent, small meals.
* Eat plenty of carbohydrate foods, which are easy to digest, provide energy, and spare protein.
* Avoid greasy or spicy foods, rich foods, and foods with a great deal of butter or fat.
* Put crackers, popcorn, dry cereal, or vanilla wafers in a plastic bag next to your bed. Eat something when you wake up but before you get up. This starts the digestive processes that will remove excess acid from your stomach and relieve the nausea. Have your breakfast after the nausea subsides.
* Get up slowly—sudden movement can aggravate nausea.
* Be sure you have fresh air in the room where you sleep.
* Avoid cooking odors; let your mate fix his own breakfast, and breakfast for the rest of the family.
* Take iron supplements only as directed. If they upset your stomach, ask your doctor if you can delay taking them for a few weeks.
* Do not drink beverages or soup with meals, but be sure to get enough liquids between meals, especially if you are vomiting. Fruit juice and carbonated beverages are easy to digest and will supply some needed carbohydrates if you are having difficulty keeping down foods.
* What makes one woman sick is soothing to another woman. Foods commonly experienced as either very good or very bad are milk and tea. Most women find cold foods and beverages easier to take than hot foods.
* Eat a high-protein snack before bed to stabilize blood sugar. A small glass of apple juice or other fruit juice

when you wake up may restore blood sugar levels and relieve nausea.

* Limit coffee because it also stimulates acid secretion. Even the smell of coffee can have this effect.
* Stop smoking. Smoking increases secretion of stomach acid, which can cause nausea.
* Listen to your body; do whatever seems to work for you.

*Medications* should be avoided if at all possible, but many physicians prescribe *Bendectin* for nausea and vomiting during pregnancy. Over 30 million women worldwide have taken Bendectin since it was introduced in 1956. In September 1980, the Fertility and Maternal Health Drug Advisory Committee

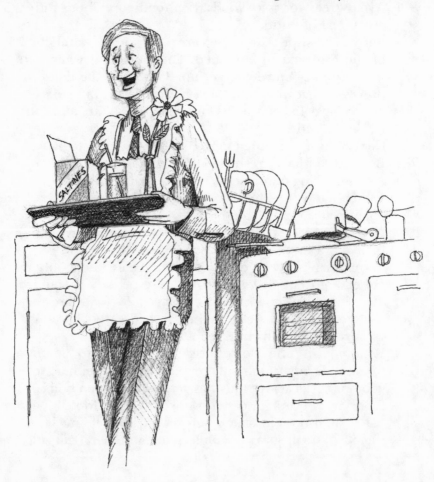

advised the FDA that Bendectin should be used only where "significant" nausea and vomiting was unresponsive to conservative treatment, such as dietary control.[98] Studies conducted early in 1982 show Bendectin to be quite safe and effective.

In response to a question about using Vitamin $B_6$, Dr. Jean Mayer and registered dietitian Jeanne Goldberg responded in their syndicated newspaper column, "Pyridoxine ($B_6$) has been mentioned as a treatment for nausea and vomiting of early pregnancy with only varying degrees of enthusiasm. Perhaps the most valid comment is that there really have been no well-controlled studies which demonstrate it to be effective. The newest edition of the *Recommended Dietary Allowances*, which finds insufficient evidence to justify recommending a supplement, sets the pyridoxine requirement in pregnancy at 2.6 milligrams a day, just 0.6 milligrams above normal."[107]

Be sure to include foods containing adequate $B_6$ in your diet, but do not take vitamin supplements for morning sickness without a doctor's prescription. Taking one of the B vitamins alone can upset the balance and utilization of other vitamins. The need for $B_6$ (pyridoxine) can be met by following the Nutritional Game Plan, Chapter 7. Dr. Mayer also says, "If you like it and are accustomed to using it, yeast is an excellent source."[107]

*Caution*: Though you may fear that you will lose the baby if you are vomiting severely, this is not likely. Nor will vomiting early in pregnancy have a negative effect on the birth weight of your baby.[73] The more immediate danger is that if you cannot eat, you will not provide nutrients to the baby, and may risk dehydration from loss of fluids.

---

**INFORM YOUR DOCTOR IF:**
* You are vomiting and unable to keep down fluids.
* You vomit more than twice a day.
* You are still experiencing nausea and vomiting after your fourteenth week of pregnancy.

---

### Constipation/Frequent Urination

Everyday toilet routines become an important part of your life when you are pregnant! Somehow these biological functions seem to give most women problems. *Many of the bowel and bladder problems can be solved by simple dietary changes. Avoid the over-the-counter remedies you may have used before pregnancy.*

*Cause*: There are two factors that impair bowel and bladder functioning when you are pregnant:

1. The uterus grows and puts pressure on your bladder and intestines.
2. Hormones of pregnancy slow the muscle action of the intestines.

The expansion of the uterus begins early in pregnancy, causing the sensation of a full bladder—one of the early signs of pregnancy. As food passes more slowly through the stomach and intestines, maximum amounts of nutrients and fluids are extracted. The food mass is moved along slowly by smooth muscles that have been relaxed by hormones produced from the beginning of pregnancy. The result can be irregularity, constipation, and maybe hemorrhoids.

*Treatment*: The best treatment is *prevention*.
* Constipation can be reduced by drinking plenty of liquids —at least eight glasses a day.
* Eat high-fiber foods (dried and fresh fruits, bran cereals, whole grains, raw vegetables) that help hold water in the stool.
* Eat prunes or figs or drink prune juice. These fruits contain isatin, a natural laxative.

Also, get some *exercise* each day to keep things moving along. If you do become constipated, *do not take laxatives* unless they are prescribed by your doctor. Mineral oil inhibits vitamin and mineral absorption and should be avoided. Your doctor may prescribe a stool softener instead of a laxative. Or try one of the old-fashioned remedies that still works: a glass of warm water with lemon juice in it, or prune juice. Your physician may make an adjustment in your iron supplement prescription if it is aggravating the situation.

You may be bothered by the frequent need to urinate. Not

surprising, considering that your bladder is being pushed, kicked, and shoved. It is also being pressed into ever-tighter quarters by your growing uterus. Some exercises, including several taught in Lamaze and other childbirth classes, may improve the muscle tone of the bladder.

Many women need a rest-room "pit stop" mid-meal, after a meal, and then an hour later. There is really nothing that can be done about this. Drinking less fluid during the evening hours may allow you to sleep through at least half of the night! While you are resting, especially at the later stages of pregnancy, lie on your side so that the uterus is not pressing on blood vessels to the kidneys and inhibiting the kidneys from working properly.[171]

### Hemorrhoids

When Anne was asked to participate in a consumer research group several years ago, one of the subjects on the agenda was hemorrhoids. The group—all women—was reluctant to discuss it at first. When they finally got going, it turned out that about 75 percent of them had experienced hemorrhoids at one time or another—many during pregnancy.

"That was when I first encountered hemorrhoids," Anne recalls. "I didn't even know what they were! When the doctor explained that they were a form of varicose veins, they seemed more socially acceptable!"

*Cause*: The increased size of the uterus puts pressure on the veins in your rectum. They sometimes protrude in and around the anus.

*Treatment*:
* Avoid constipation.
* Avoid straining during elimination.
* Lie down with your rectum high, in knee-to-chest position, and apply ice packs.
* Itching and burning may be relieved by topical ointments (such as petroleum jelly) that coat the inflamed tissues. Ask your physician to recommend a suppository that is safe for you to use.

### Heartburn

*Cause*: Heartburn typically occurs during the last three months of pregnancy when your baby is growing and pushing on the surrounding organs. As your food attempts its normal downward route, the expanding uterus compresses the stomach and digested food and stomach fluids are pushed back into your esophagus, causing a feeling of pressure and burning. Although it is called heartburn, it has nothing to do with your heart.

Mary Baim said, "During the last four months, I finally learned the meaning of heartburn. I suffered, suffered, suffered—day in and day out. I carried Rolaids as if they were my house keys. It lowered the fire's flame, but never put it out."

*Treatment*:
* Relax and eat slowly.
* Do not overeat at any meal; eat several small meals instead.
* Avoid highly seasoned, rich, fatty, and fried foods.
* If a specific food bothers you, avoid it until after you deliver.
* Wear comfortable, loose-fitting clothes without belts.
* Do not lie down flat after you eat. If you wish to rest, prop your back and head on pillows. Walk around to encourage the gastric juices to flow down, not up.
* If you have heartburn at night, elevate your head and shoulders with pillows.
* Never take antacids without a doctor's specific direction to do so. In pregnancy, a suggestion or prescription may be given for a medication containing aluminum hydroxide gel, magnesium trisilicate, or magnesium hydroxide. *Do not take medications containing sodium bicarbonate* (baking soda), which prevents absorption of important vitamins and minerals. Some (such as Alka-Seltzer) have large amounts of sodium that may promote fluid retention in your body tissues (edema).

## Aches, Pains, Cramps

*Cause*: There are all sorts of little pains, and sometimes not so little pains, especially during the last weeks of pregnancy. Most are caused by pressure of the growing baby on your stomach, bladder, nerves, intestines, ribs, lungs, and what sometimes seems like every muscle and bone in your body. The baby is getting ready to break loose!

Anne's youngest daughter, Mary, has always been a very athletic child. "I think she did calisthenics in the womb, and she was constantly kicking me! I used to shove her to get her to move over and leave my poor aching ribs alone. To this day, she cannot sit still for long."

Muscle cramps in the legs and abdomen are frequent, especially at night when you are tired. Muscle cramps have been related to an imbalance of calcium and phosphorus, but studies have failed to confirm this.

*Treatment*: Your doctor may want to reduce the phosphorus in the diet to control muscle cramps. There are several ways to do this. Anything that will increase circulation will increase leg cramps.

Methods of treating muscle cramps include lying or sitting down and elevating your legs, or pressing your foot against a hard surface if the pain is in your foot. Rapid, firm massaging while moving the foot up and down reduces the cramp, but the leg or foot may continue to hurt for some time. Exercise, particularly walking, is helpful.

## Edema—Not Such a Swell Thing

Some degree of swelling during the last trimester of pregnancy is normal, and should not be confused with the kind of edema that accompanies nonpregnant conditions. In a study of twenty-four thousand women in Aberdeen, Scotland, Dr. F. E. Hytten, a physician who documented many of the physiological changes of pregnancy, found that edema was associated with better reproductive performance.[47]

*Cause*: The same hormones that cause some women to retain water in their bodies just before they menstruate cause water retention during pregnancy. Connective tissues become more elastic during the last months of pregnancy, and "reservoirs" of water form in your ankles, hands, legs, and so on. These water-filled cells help hold your expanded blood volume during pregnancy, offset losses that occur during delivery, and contribute to the production of breast milk. Meanwhile, you will probably be more comfortable if you buy a pair of shoes a size bigger than your usual size!

Most of this fluid is lost during delivery but some edema may remain after the baby is born. The remaining fluid is usually excreted during the week after delivery as the hormonal balance shifts.[148] Some women, as hormones and fluids shift, actually develop edema after delivery for a few days.[160]

*Treatment*: Until recently, doctors routinely advised salt restriction and diuretics (water pills) to relieve edema. Current medical research, however, advises:

* *Do not take diuretics.*
* Do not limit salt—use salt on foods "to taste."
* Since swelling in your legs and feet is aggravated by the pressure of the uterus as it presses on your veins, rest on your left side with your feet up four or five times a day. This permits better return circulation of blood from your legs.
* Wear comfortable shoes that allow your feet to expand.
* Remove tight rings.
* Some excess water may be held in tissues because the growing baby is blocking normal flow to the kidneys. Lie on your side to allow the kidneys to work more efficiently when you sleep.

The movement of fluids in and out of cells is essential to maintain your expanded blood volume. The delicate balance can be upset if you take diuretics, which remove fluids and sodium by increasing urination. Use of diuretics can cause nausea, vomiting, headache, and loss of appetite. They should be used only in special situations determined by your doctor.

## Anemia

The problem with anemia is that many women think they have it and they do not, and many women do not think they have it and they do! You are not anemic just because you feel tired. The only way to know if you are anemic is to have a blood test and this is done routinely early in pregnancy. When you are pregnant, it makes a big difference—so find out!

There are two types of nutritional anemia that are prevalent during pregnancy. Many women enter pregnancy critically affected by *iron deficiency* and as many as 25 percent develop *low levels of folacin* (*folic acid,* one of the B vitamins) during their pregnancy.[100]

*Cause*:

* You may have entered pregnancy with anemia due to poor dietary intake of these blood-forming nutrients.
* You may have regularly taken medications that interfere with absorption. Oral contraceptives can interfere with folacin utilization; antacids can interfere with iron absorption.
* You may have depleted levels because you have had a recent pregnancy or are carrying more than one baby.
* As soon as you become pregnant, your needs for iron and folacin dramatically increase. Your expanded blood volume requires iron; rapid fetal cell-division and growth doubles your need for folacin. Your baby depends on your diet to build up reserves of iron for the first six months after birth.
* You may not be taking your prescribed supplements regularly.

*Treatment:*

* Eat plenty of foods rich in iron and folacin.
* Your doctor will prescribe supplements to correct existing deficiencies.

Folacin and iron are discussed in Chapters 5 and 6.

### Beyond Self-Help

Up to this point, the problems described, if not abnormally severe, can be treated by diet modification, exercise, or relief methods that you can manage on your own. Of course, you will want to tell your doctor, but generally you can manage the control measures.

There are, however, nutrition-related complications during pregnancy that require careful medical monitoring and supervision, and dietary modification beyond the scope of this book, and perhaps beyond the care that can be given by your regular physician.

If you encounter complications such as those described in the following pages, you will want to seek information about current treatments, specialists, and facilities available in your area. We offer some explanation only so that you will know what to expect. What was possible or dangerous only a few years ago is now considered almost routine because there are so many obstetricians and gynecologists with special medical and technical skills who can care for women with complicated pregnancies.

Not too many years ago, women with diabetes or other chronic diseases were advised not to bear children. Now many of these women can, and do, have healthy children. But each must know that it will be a difficult nine months, both physically and emotionally. *Good medical management, a nutritious diet, and plenty of rest give you the best chance of having a healthy baby. The advances of modern science make possible many babies that are truly miracles.*

### Diabetes Mellitus

In *The Baby Team*, diabetes is described this way:
"Insulin is a substance, or hormone, produced by an organ called the pancreas. We depend on insulin to help sugar, or glucose, travel from the bloodstream into many of the tissues of the body where it is used for energy. Diabetes is a condition in which not enough insulin is produced, utilized or released by the pancreas to do this job. As a consequence, sugar is 'trapped' in the bloodstream and cannot get to the tissues. When we

measure the amount of sugar in the blood of a diabetic, we find that it is higher than normal. This potential energy is 'wasted' in urine."[9]

If your doctor suspects diabetes, you will be given a glucose tolerance test. Your doctor will advise you to eat nothing after dinner the night before the test, and to come in the morning without eating breakfast. Blood samples will be taken before you eat, and at various times after you drink a special sugar-water solution or eat a meal with a measured amount of sugar.

The blood tests will show the rate at which your blood sugar rises after eating sugar, and the rate of insulin release that returns the blood sugar to a "normal" level. If your blood sugar does not return to the "normal" range within a certain time, you may have diabetes mellitus.

Pregnancy is a time when known diabetes becomes more severe and when previously unsuspected diabetes is more likely to appear. During the second half of pregnancy, hormones are produced by the placenta that oppose the action of insulin. This creates an extra demand on the pancreas to produce more insulin. If it cannot, diabetes occurs.

If you are diabetic, you will need to know that:

1. A controlled diet is essential to the management of diabetes and can reduce the incidence and severity of many of the symptoms and complications. A diet will be devised just for you based on your specific habits and needs. Although almost all of the information in this book is applicable, the specific number of servings and types of food must be modified to meet your individual needs, with frequent reassessments as the pregnancy progresses.
2. Several complications of pregnancy are more common in women who have diabetes. These include pre-eclampsia (described later in this chapter), excessive fluid surrounding the baby, and prematurity. Complications of diabetes are sometimes intensified during pregnancy. These include changes in the retina of the eye and in the kidney.[9]
3. Diabetes is a high-risk situation in pregnancy. Care of a

pregnant woman with diabetes requires full knowledge of the altered metabolism of both pregnancy and diabetes. It can be very tricky business and is one of the situations that require strict medical management. Control of blood sugar levels is a very important part of your care and must be used in conjunction with good medical management to produce a healthy normal baby. Very high, or very low, levels of your blood sugar can be dangerous to your baby.

The doctor can often detect early signs of problems or potential complications. Find a good doctor because you will see him/her often. Keep all of your medical appointments and do not hesitate to call with questions or problems.

Two types of diabetes occur during pregnancy:

1. *Diabetes existing before pregnancy and remaining after delivery.*

Most women with this form of diabetes know they have it, have been treating it with insulin and/or diet, and will continue to have it after delivery. If you are a diabetic in this category, discuss the implications of pregnancy with your doctor before you stop birth-control measures and attempt to become pregnant. The physician who helps you manage your diabetes may recommend an obstetrician who will treat you during your pregnancy, or with whom she can work to supervise your care. The specific plan of care will be based on the duration of your diabetes, existing complications, and your physical and emotional needs.

You should expect to strictly control your food intake and the sugar levels in your blood and urine. Your diet and medications will have to be changed many times throughout your pregnancy as your hormonal levels shift and the baby grows. You are likely to be hospitalized for careful blood-sugar monitoring at the beginning and at times during your pregnancy, and the baby may be delivered a bit earlier than your due date. If you want to breastfeed, you can, but will need guidance from a registered dietitian or your physician and yet another dietary modification.

2. *Diabetes that begins during pregnancy—and disappears after delivery.*

From 1 to 3 percent of all pregnant women—thirty thousand to ninety thousand women each year in this country —become diabetic during their pregnancies.[67] It usually occurs during the latter half of pregnancy, when there is an increased need for insulin production. This *gestational diabetes* generally disappears after the baby's birth, though 60 percent of those who have it develop diabetes later in life.[67]

If tests for levels of sugar in the blood or urine show that you have gestational diabetes, the obstetrician may recommend that you be evaluated by an internist, diabetologist, or endocrinologist. All of these medical specialties have additional training in the management of pregnant women with diabetes. Some obstetricians prefer to manage the gestational diabetic more directly—for this form of diabetes is usually less difficult to control and generally has fewer complications than insulin-dependent diabetes.

Harriet was diagnosed a gestational diabetic. A tiny dynamo who entered her pregnancies at less than one hundred pounds, she had no family history of diabetes. When her obstetrician discovered she had diabetes, he referred Harriet to an internist who specialized in diabetes. She was given a diet pattern and food lists and was able to manage her diabetes without oral medications or insulin. When it was determined that the baby was big enough, Harriet had a Cesarean section. Laura weighed 7 pounds, 9 ounces, and was perfectly healthy. Harriet's diabetes was gone when she left the hospital.

The same situation occurred during her pregnancy with Karen two years later. Harriet knows that she may become diabetic at some time in her life. Laura is now thirteen and there is no indication of diabetes in either mother or children.

In recent years, great advances have been made in caring for the pregnant diabetic and her baby. Most gestational diabetics are now allowed to carry their babies the full nine months.

There are a number of resources that provide guidance to the diabetic woman who is considering having a baby or who is already pregnant. Call your local affiliate chapter of the American Diabetes Association and ask for the information they have available on diabetes in pregnancy. One of their publications, *Diabetes Forecast*, has a number of excellent articles on the subject.

Also, there is a wonderful book, written by a physician and a nurse who is a diabetic, called *The Baby Team*, by Donald R. Coustan, M.D., and Sheila Garvey, R.N. Its subtitle tells it all: "A Positive Approach to Pregnancy with Diabetes." It costs $2.50 and it is available from Monoject, Division of Sherwood Medical Department, T.I., 1831 Olive Street, St. Louis, MO 63103.

For an explanation of the diabetic diet and how food should be prepared for diabetics, refer to *The Art of Cooking for the Diabetic* by Katharine Middleton and Mary Abbott Hess. It was published by Contemporary Books in 1978, and is available as a Signet paperback in most bookstores. Not only are the recipes some of our favorites, but all are calculated for use by diabetics and each recipe explains how it can be modified if your diet also restricts salt.

### Hypertension

Hypertension is the medical term for *high blood pressure*. Like sugar in your urine, high blood pressure is a sign that something is not working as it should. Because there are several types of hypertension that can occur during pregnancy, your doctor will want to determine the *reason* before suggesting *treatment*.

Many women in this country, especially low-income black women, suffer from hypertension during their childbirth years.[46] Some have it and know they have it before they become pregnant; others find out when their blood pressure is taken at the doctor's office. Some may develop hypertension as the result of problems directly related to pregnancy. Regardless of its cause, elevations in blood pressure must be treated to avoid endangering either you or your baby! Rest will be absolutely essential, combined with careful medical monitoring.

### Toxemia

Toxemia is not what a lot of people think it is. It is *not* the inevitable result of gaining more than average weight. It is *not* caused by retaining water or eating foods with too much salt. It is *not* what its name suggests it to be: "Tox" (poison) and "emia" (blood).

What toxemia *is* is one of the most controversial areas of obstetrical research.[57] Many researchers suggest that nutrition plays a major role; others argue that nutrition is not a direct cause.

In the United States, toxemia occurs most frequently in women with very low incomes. Some believe the reason is that these women are often poorly nourished. These women usually get less prenatal care and have a higher rate of obstetrical complications.

There have been consistent reports that toxemia (especially among poorly nourished women) is reduced when calories and protein are increased. Agnes Higgins of the Montreal Diet Dispensary has used this technique with impressive results.[175] Her evidence suggests that toxemia can be prevented by improved diets. However, Leon Chesley, Ph.D., one of the most respected authorities on the subject, reviewed data on wartime mothers whose diets were extremely limited. He found that there was no significant increase in the incidence of toxemia.[5]

In addition to low income and poor diets, both before and during pregnancy, statistics point toward other risk factors. Women who are most likely to develop toxemia are those who:

* have mothers or sisters who developed toxemia in their first pregnancy.
* are in their first pregnancy; toxemia is less common in later pregnancies.
* are carrying twins (or more than one baby).
* are in their first pregnancy and are less than twenty years of age, or are thirty-five years or older.
* have existing high blood pressure, kidney disease, or diabetes, or have inadequate medical care.[133]

It is generally agreed that weight gain of over 30 pounds is not a factor. This figure, which was once believed to be the uppermost amount that a woman could safely gain, is now considered well within normal limits. In fact, early work by Dr. Winslow T. Tompkins, a pioneer in research on maternal nutritional status in the first half of this century, found an increased incidence of toxemia among women who were *under-weight* at conception and failed to gain enough weight during their pregnancy.[138] Thus part of the dilemma of toxemia may be the duration of poor nutritional status as well as actual food consumed during the pregnancy.

Chesley's excellent comprehensive review of many of the suggested theories related to toxemia concludes that the cause of toxemia is unknown.[5]

Toxemia occurs in escalating degrees of seriousness:

1. *Pre-eclampsia.* General edema including fluid retention in the hands and face, high blood pressure (hypertension), and protein in the urine.[137] A weight gain of over 2 pounds in one week is an indication of potential pre-eclampsia in the last trimester. Bedrest, a good diet, and medical care may arrest the situation, but hospitalization may be necessary. In pre-eclampsia, there is a significant decrease in blood flow to the placenta. Bedrest may improve the situation.
2. *Eclampsia.* If pre-eclampsia goes untreated, convulsions may occur; *this* is eclampsia. Danger signs are blurred vision, a headache, or abdominal pain. If any of these signs occurs, call your doctor immediately. Both you and your baby may be in extreme danger.

We wish that we could say that if you ate a balanced diet, you could prevent toxemia. Unfortunately, we cannot. While more women from the lower socio-economic classes have toxemia, some middle-class women have also developed it. Toxemia during pregnancy remains the subject of much speculation and medical debate.

If you are eating a nutritious diet, following the advice in this book, and getting good prenatal care, you are doing everything that you can do to prevent toxemia, based on what is known at this time.

## Heart or Kidney Disease

Women with diseases of the heart or kidneys are included in the high-risk group that require specialized care. Pregnancy makes increased demands on the heart and kidney, which are not functioning normally. Heart disease is the one situation where a low-sodium diet plays a major role in medical management of pregnancy. Your care must be closely supervised by medical specialists. Rest and dietary modifications will surely be parts of the plan, customized for your individual physiological problems.

We hope that the information in this book helps you to understand the dietary modifications that may be necessary, and will motivate you to comply so that you will provide for maximum health and well-being for yourself and your baby.

There are many other medical problems that can occur during pregnancy that do not have specific dietary implications. We do not want to minimize the necessity for care for them. But this book deals specifically with nutrition and pregnancy.

# 10.
# Breast or Bottle:
# A Big Decision

How do you intend to feed your baby in the first few months of life? "Breast is best!" say nutrition-conscious health professionals. Even the makers of formulas concede the superiority of mother's milk.

In 1978, both the American Academy of Pediatrics and the Canadian Pediatric Society officially endorsed breast feeding as the preferred method of infant feeding. They called mother's milk "the best food for every newborn infant," and recommended that physicians urge all mothers to breastfeed their infants for the first four to six months of life. The American Medical Association and the American Public Health Association also have position papers endorsing breastfeeding.

Observations show that breastfed babies are generally healthier during their first year of life. Respiratory and digestive disorders are much more common in bottle-fed babies; they have more visits to the doctor for various illnesses.

Breastfeeding reduces the inclination to overfeed the baby.

While bottle-fed babies may be encouraged to "empty the bottle," the breastfed baby will stop sucking when satisfied. Overfeeding during infancy has been correlated with obesity during childhood and even adult life.[15]

Possibly the most significant difference between breast milk and formula is that breast milk contains a variety of substances that protect the baby from disease and speed development of the baby's defense systems. Human milk contains many immunity carriers, antibodies, and infection-fighters called "macrophages" that protect the infant's digestive tract from bacteria and allergies. Many of these "Big Macs" have only recently been discovered; there is a variety of other protectors known and probably some not yet discovered. These factors are not present in cow's milk or prepared formula.

In another time and place, there would be no choice—you would do as all mothers did, and breastfeed your baby. Today, in Third World countries where sanitation, a safe water supply, refrigeration, and money to buy infant formula are severely limited, bottle-feeding is still not a viable option.

In our country, however, most babies can grow and thrive on either breast or bottle milk. If the decision about what to feed your baby was being made only on the basis of the nutritional composition of the milk and its immune properties, there would be little question as to your choice; the reality is that the decision is influenced by a number of other factors.

*Your authors have healthy children—some fed by bottle, others by breast, but all nourished with love and care, which, we feel, is what matters most. We have had good experiences with both methods of feeding.*

*Decide how you will feed your baby while you are pregnant. Discuss it with those who are close to you during your pregnancy.* Disagreements about feeding during the emotionally fragile days following delivery can be upsetting. A new mother needs support in caring for her baby, not criticism. Your decision can influence your choice of physician, types of medication used during delivery, and even the hospital. Regardless of which way you choose to feed your baby, you will need to know what to expect so you can make the necessary preparations.

*This chapter will give you the information so that you can decide.* It is not instructional: we will not go into the preparation of formula or the physiology of breastfeeding, or deal with problems that may develop. That information is available in other sources and from your obstetrician and pediatrician. This book deals with your pregnancy and decisions and actions during this time, not after your baby is born.

You may already have decided how you want to feed your baby. Some women choose to bottle-feed because this is what their friends have done. If you are a working woman, and intend to return to work shortly after the baby is born, you may think breastfeeding is not possible. You may not have considered nursing because you do not know much about it, do not know anyone who has done it, and frankly, are a little afraid to try it. You may not want to risk being disappointed if you aren't able to nurse. If you tried unsuccessfully to nurse a child before, you may assume that you cannot nurse this child either. There are many reasons. . . .

Just ten years ago, far more American women chose to bottle-feed their babies. Now, so many women have been convinced by the arguments in favor of breast-feeding that there has been a radical increase in breastfeeding in the United States. More than 50 percent of new mothers are now doing it, and 23 percent are still at it five or six months later![80] The incidence of breastfeeding is higher on the West Coast than the East Coast, and higher in women with more years of formal education.[167]

Many first-time mothers today have little idea of what is involved in either breast- or bottle-feeding an infant. There was a time when most women of childbearing age had grown up in extended families where there were babies, and they picked up a lot of knowhow. Today's young mother may have had little exposure to infants. She may never have seen a baby being nursed or prepared a formula. She may not have any idea about what constitutes a "normal" feeding pattern. You may find yourself being faced with making a decision about something about which you know very little.

Whatever your thoughts, you will feel better about your decision if you examine the pros and cons of both breast- and bottle-feeding, and choose what is right for you.

## Milk for Human Babies

Milk is a product of evolution, designed specifically to nourish the offspring of mammals during the delicate period after leaving the womb.

The same nutrients are present in the milk of all mammals, but the composition of each is different. Mother's milk is designed to meet the specific needs of the species. The baby whale, for example, has enormous energy needs, but he cannot stay under water for long periods of time to nurse. His mother's milk is very concentrated, and a little takes the baby a long way. Human babies, on the other hand, because they grow slowly, do not need great quantities of nutrients; they thrive on frequent, small feedings.

Both breast and bottle provide adequate calories for the first four months. Addition of solid foods before four months of age may result in too many calories being consumed. There is no evidence that early introduction of solid foods will pacify a fussy baby. Statistics show that by *one week*, almost 20 percent of infants in the United States are being given some solid foods; by one month, the figure jumps to 90 percent.[144] The early addition of solid foods is often at the request of the mother. It is not in the best interest of the baby.

Like any other food, milk can be broken down into its components: carbohydrate, fat, protein, vitamins, minerals, and water. Scientists can actually write a recipe or "formula" for human milk, listing the amount of each ingredient. Cow's milk can be modified to meet the specifications by adding and subtracting various components. Many infant formulas now on the market have a base made from soybeans instead of cow's milk. The quality and composition of formula never varies and the quantity being fed is evident.

Human milk varies in composition from mother to mother, day to day, morning to night, first minute of feeding to last, from one meal the mother eats to the next and on the quality of the mother's diet. It is very difficult to assess individual variations in the volume of milk produced. Some babies drink far more than the "average" production of 850 milliliters (3½ cups) of breast milk each day.[18] Recommended standards of

nutrient intake for lactating women are based on the level of
nutrients excreted in a *standard* amount of milk. So while you
may be able to produce good-quality milk, it is hard to
determine precisely what level of dietary intake will produce
*enough* milk for an especially hungry baby.

The following chart compares the "real thing" and the
"made from recipe" bottled alternative.

## A COMPARISON OF HUMAN MILK AND BABY FORMULA

### HUMAN MILK

### BABY FORMULA

#### Calories

The total number of calories from fat
are about the same in human and
cow's milk; however, only 10% of
calories in human milk is from protein, and 40% is from carbohydrate.

In cow's milk 50% of calories are
divided evenly between protein and
carbohydrate. Cow's-milk–based
formulas are diluted and fortified
with carbohydrate to yield a product
similar in caloric values to breast
milk. Has about twenty calories per
ounce.

#### Carbohydrate

The main type of carbohydrate in
human milk is lactose. Human milk
tastes sweeter than cow's milk.

Lactose creates acidity in the baby's
intestinal tract, which discourages
many kinds of bacteria that can
cause disease.

Lactose is broken down into glucose
and galactose, which are easily
absorbed.

Lactose increases calcium
absorption.

Lactose or other carbohydrates are
added to formulas to approximate
human milk sugar content.

## HUMAN MILK                    BABY FORMULA

### Protein

Human milk has a relatively low protein content, but the protein is well utilized. It is adequate to meet the protein needs of the baby until age six months; from six to eleven months, ¾ of the child's protein need can be supplied from breast milk.[55]

Cow's milk contains about twice as much protein as human milk, but the protein is not absorbed as well as that of breast milk. Ready-to-use formula has been modified to provide the proper concentration.

The type of protein in human milk is easily digested. The sweet smell associated with breastfed babies and the lack of odor in their stool, urine, and regurgitated milk indicates that the digestion and absorption of the protein and fat is relatively complete.[16]

Mixing formula concentrate according to directions is essential to provide the proper amount of protein.

Breast milk contains anti-infective proteins that are absent in cow's milk. Human milk lacks beta-lactoglobulin, the most common cause of allergic reactions to cow's milk. Human milk is the best protection against food allergies in infancy.[163]

Immunizing factors are less essential for the survival of healthy babies born in the United States where the water supply is safe and there is less exposure to diseases.

The amino-acid patterns in human milk and cow's milk are very different; because of this, human milk is better for premature or low-birth-weight babies. Human milk contains large amounts of taurine, an amino acid needed for brain growth. The role of taurine in the developing baby is just being explored.[50]
The milk of a woman who gives birth prematurely may be higher in protein than the milk of a mother who carries to term. This is just what a premature baby needs to thrive.[173]

Infant formulas are now available that meet specific amino-acid needs, such as those required by premature babies.

# HUMAN MILK

# BABY FORMULA

## Fat

The type of fat in human milk is influenced by the mother's diet. If her diet is low in fat, her milk will reflect the reserves of fat in her body, which are then utilized to make the milk.

Breast milk contains a substance that aids in rapid digestion and absorption of human milk fat.[16]

Human milk fat is predominantly unsaturated and polyunsaturated.

Human milk contains more cholesterol than cow's milk. New research indicates that cholesterol in human milk may induce enzymes that better utilize cholesterol later in life.[50] Studies show that cholesterol may play a role in preventing infections in babies.[104]

"Hind milk," which comes in near the end of feeding, has more fat than milk at the beginning of the feeding, contributing to the baby's feeling of fullness, which limits intake.

Different mothers have different amounts of fat in their milk. Observations of expressed breast milks show that some look more like skim milk, while other samples look very creamy.[176]

Many formulas replace saturated butterfat in cow's milk with unsaturated and polyunsaturated vegetable oils. Soy-based formulas do not contain saturated fat.

| HUMAN MILK | BABY FORMULA |
|---|---|

## VITAMINS

| | |
|---|---|
| All the vitamins required for good nutrition and health can be supplied in breast milk, with the possible exception of vitamin D.[144] | Most formulas are fortified with vitamins to ensure adequate nutrients for the baby. |
| Babies who are not routinely exposed to sunlight, because of their environment, who have dark skin, or because they have been covered in clothing that blocks light from the body, are often given supplementary vitamin D in addition to breast milk. Recently a water-soluble vitamin D has been isolated in breast milk, but the degree to which it is utilized is, as yet, unknown. | Virtually all formulas are fortified with vitamin D. |
| The quantity of water-soluble vitamins in breast milk is determined by the mother's intake of these vitamins. | |
| Breast milk does not pass along adequate vitamin K until the fourth day after birth. For this reason, many newborns are given supplements to protect them against postnatal hemorrhages. | Vitamin K is routinely given to newborns. |

## MINERALS

| | |
|---|---|
| Mineral concentration is less than in cow's milk, but presumably this is easier for the newborn to handle than the more concentrated minerals in cow's milk. | The concentration of minerals in cow's milk is much greater than in breast milk. Infant formulas have been adjusted to lower this concentration so that it is more like human milk. |

### (Sodium)

| | |
|---|---|
| There is less sodium in human milk than in cow's milk. | Cow's milk contains three to four times the amount of sodium than is in human milk, but when salt was removed from a formula several years ago, some chloride deficiencies developed, so it was restored. |

## HUMAN MILK

## BABY FORMULA

### (Fluoride)

Little fluoride is passed from the mother to the baby in her milk. While the La Leche League does not recommend supplements to breastfed babies, many health professionals prescribe 25 milligrams/day to infants, especially if they do not have supplementary bottles of water.[167] Some health professionals question the value of supplements because fluoride is most effective if administered over a period of time, as in drinking water, not in a single dose.[173]

Formulas (which come in concentrated form) contain very low levels of fluoride to prevent overdoses in areas where the formula is mixed with fluoridated water. If the formula is made with unfluoridated water, a supplement of 25 milligrams/day may be prescribed.

### (Zinc)

There is a high concentration of zinc in colostrum, the first milk that comes after delivery; then the amount drops off and relatively low levels are maintained. The amount normally present is apparently adequate, however, because breastfed babies do not experience zinc deficiencies. There are zinc-binding factors in human milk that increase absorption.[163]

Level is similar to human milk, but absorption rate is low. If a deficiency develops, 35 milligrams of zinc a day, given orally, will cure it.[163]

### (Iron)

Human milk contains little iron, but this is not generally a problem if the mother has had adequate iron during pregnancy to allow the fetus to build up reserves that last during

Babies fed unfortified formula can develop anemia at about four months. Babies given iron-fortified formula rarely become anemic.

## A COMPARISON OF HUMAN MILK
## AND BABY FORMULA *(cont.)*

## HUMAN MILK                    BABY FORMULA

### (Iron)

his first few months after birth. Premature babies may not have had a
chance to build up adequate reserves, and must receive iron supplements.

The iron content of breast milk is low,
but the absorption rate is high, and
breastfed babies rarely, if ever, become iron-deficient.[144]

Babies who are being breastfed
should not be given supplementary
foods during the first four months of
life, as these may affect iron absorption. After that time, they will need
iron from fortified cereals and other
iron-rich foods.[120]

### (Calcium and Phosphorus)

The baby receives calcium in breast       There are much higher levels of cal-
milk even when the mother does not        cium and phosphorus in cow's milk.
consume adequate calcium, but             The concentration is reduced by
some is drawn from her bones.[80]         diluting cow's milk in formula.

The ratio of calcium to phosphorous
is ideal for maximum mineral utilization.

In 1980, the FDA passed new laws to ensure that every
precaution be taken to make infant formula safe. *The number of
healthy children in this country who have been bottle-fed is a testimony
to the effectiveness of substitute formulas and the manner in which they
are tested to safeguard the health of infants.*

The human milk of well-nourished mothers is used as the
standard to determine the adequacy of infant formula substitutes. Modern technology has made great strides in formulat-
ing human-milk substitutes.

There are, however, some factors we cannot know for sure. While no ill-effects are currently recognized, we do not know the long-term effects of substances that are added to formulas, such as emulsifiers, thickening agents, antioxidants, and pH adjusters. In addition, there may be properties in human milk that have not yet been discovered that may not be adequately supplied in formula substitutes.

No infant-formula manufacturer has yet to fool Mother Nature. Scientific facts from a wide spectrum of disciplines have made an impact on health professionals who now are questioning the assumption that modern formulas are essentially equivalent to mother's milk. Dr. Derrick B. Jelliffe, in an article for the *New England Journal of Medicine*, stated: "In any part of the world, no single pediatric measure has such widespread and dramatic potential for child health as a return to breast feeding. Awareness of this fact seems gradually to be dawning."[97]

## A Time to Hold, a Time to Love

The most enthusiastic proponents of breastfeeding are women who have successfully nursed their children. Some may be almost *too* enthusiastic! The reason is that for many, it is an extremely emotional—and physically exciting—experience.

*Anne*: "Writing about breastfeeding for this chapter brought back all kinds of feelings. At first, it was very strange—and not always wonderful. No one told me that I would be in pain *after* the baby was born: the episiotomy hurt, my breasts were hot and tender, my nipples were sensitive, and I got very little sleep. But the feeling of the milk let-down—that tingling sensation—is one I'll never forget. The reality of the baby close to me as I held her overwhelmed me. 'Elizabeth Anne, I will take care of you, no matter what!' I've had mixed feelings about having a child—I'd never liked children much. But, as I nursed my first child, I knew I wanted her and I wanted to accept the responsibility for nurturing her. I was doing something no one else could do. It made me feel very good about myself."

Where is Dad when all this heavy baby-mother scene is going on? Frankly, many dads find it difficult. Just when he thinks, "Darling, at last . . . ," baby is hungry. New mothers have a way of being very preoccupied with nursing, and may not be interested in sex.

Some men have difficulty dealing with breastfeeding because they see the mother's breasts only within a sexual context. The idea of fondling a milk-filled breast may be repulsive. This is not at all uncommon, and should be discussed.

A man who is understanding and supportive of his partner, during these intense first weeks, encourages her love and respect. Their sexual activity, when it does resume, will reflect the new depth of their relationship.

*Bruce*: "I was very proud of Anne because she was willing to learn how to breastfeed, stuck with it, and was a great success at it. Neither of us had any experience with breastfeeding, or were close to couples who had done it, but we read the literature and decided it was definitely worth trying."

Fatherhood, like motherhood, takes training. A man who understands and supports the breastfeeding of his child feels a sense of pride as he watches the child nursing. A woman who does not have the support of her mate and family will have a difficult time trying to nurse her child.

*Bruce*: "All this talk of fathers of breastfed babies not having to get up in the night is nonsense! When the baby cried, I'd get up and change her, then bring her into our bed to be nursed. I remember thinking, 'Anne has the easy part; she never has to get up!' Sometimes, we'd all fall asleep there in bed together."

The intense feeling of attachment Anne described above is one many mothers (and to some extent, fathers) experience. The term *bonding* has been used to define the phenomenon. It happens quite naturally when the baby is breastfed, but it is not exclusive to breastfeeding. Bonding is the result of physical contact—holding, touching, smelling, stroking, rocking, feeding. It is best "skin-on-skin," with baby cuddled against Mom and encircled in her arms. This can happen regardless of the source of feeding.

*Mary*: "Whenever I think about Rachel's birth, I remember lying on the delivery table. Dr. Ellis told me she was perfect and put her on my chest. Peter came in then, and we held hands and looked at her and stroked her. I was wheeled into another room where we spent some more time together before I was taken up to my room. Somehow, by the time I got upstairs, my concern during pregnancy (that I might not like being a mother) disappeared, and both Peter and I knew that she was ours, that we would always love her, and that we were a family. It was one of the most special times of my life. This is what 'bonding' is all about. It had nothing to do with breastfeeding, because I had chosen to bottle-feed, which was the best decision for me and my family."

Research just completed shows that there are long-term effects of bonding. A study conducted over a period of five years compared mothers and infants who had an additional sixteen hours or more of close contact during the first three days after birth with a group that did not have the extra contact. After two years, mothers in the extra-contact group seemed more interested in their children's development. They used more complex language in talking with their children and spent time explaining cause and effect.[119] Some sociologists and psychologists have written that when there are "disorders of bonding"—that is, when an opportunity for bonding does not occur—there is an increased frequency of child abuse and other behaviors that are not protective of the child.

Until recently, it was customary to separate mothers and babies after delivery, and keep the babies in a newborn nursery during the hospital stay. Fortunately, many hospitals now have *rooming in,* or some provision for mother and father (and sometimes other family members) to hold and care for the baby soon after birth. This arrangement facilitates bonding.

Talk to your doctor about this early in your pregnancy and try to plan delivery at a hospital where your baby can stay with you rather than in a separate nursery. This may not be possible because either mother or baby may need a lot of medical attention. But you won't know this until after the delivery.

Parents of both breast- and bottle-fed babies will want to make a special point of holding and cuddling their babies during these important first weeks. Men do not live by bread alone, and babies do not thrive on milk alone!

## A Time to Work, a Time to Play

One of the major factors affecting the decision to breast- or bottle-feed is the time element. Many women today return to jobs or school shortly after their baby's birth; others are active in social or community activities; some frankly admit they just do not want to be tied down to their baby.

If this is your first child, we should warn you that immediately after delivery, you are going to need some time to rest, regardless of how you decide to feed your baby. If you decide to breastfeed, the times of rest and relaxation automatically come with the nursing. You can't very well nurse the baby and do the washing at the same time. You can, however, read a book or watch television.

New babies require a great deal of time and attention. Newborn babies frequently nurse every hour and a half to three hours for periods of five to ten minutes; bottle-fed babies must be fed every three to four hours. The amount of milk they can consume at first is limited, by the size of their stomachs, to only 1 to 3 ounces. Whether a fussy baby is being offered its mother's breast, a bottle, or a pacifier, being rocked or walked, it all takes time.

A woman who has other children may find it frightening to contemplate caring for a baby in addition to her other children. You've no doubt heard it said that the first baby takes all of your time, and somehow the babies who follow just fit in. The first baby is the most time-consuming because you are learning; the subsequent children are generally easier.

*Anne*: "I was very anxious about my first child. Did she get enough to eat? What caused the rash on her chest? Was she wet? Was there a pin threatening to puncture her tiny body (that was in the good old days of real diapers)? I nursed watching the clock and taking care to start on the 'right side.' She thrived.

"Along came Jennifer, twenty-two months later. The baby proved to be a piece of cake compared to my rambunctious toddler. Poor Jennifer never got a full meal! She was nursed in fits and starts—she sometimes cried, but at least she stayed put when I laid her down. She too, thrived. To this day, she delights in attention—but seldom demands it."

Toddlers can sit near you and have a story read to them while the baby is being fed. They will enjoy the attention and feel less resentment toward the newcomer if they are included in this important task.

There was a time when the expense of feeding a baby was a viable reason to breastfeed. However, the cost of extra food to feed the mother who breastfeeds must now be considered. While there may be some women who think about cost when making their decision, it is no longer a major factor.

If you breastfeed, the preparation of food takes no time at all, and you can leave off and resume, if necessary, to meet the immediate needs of other children. The milk will be fresh and ready whenever you and your baby get together. For both day and night feedings, both the responsibility and the joy of nourishing will be yours. Other family members can hold and care for the baby at other times.

If you bottle-feed, you will have to spend some time preparing the bottles. Although most modern formulas are sterile in the can, just to be poured into clean bottles, it still takes some time. If you choose to bottle-feed, the pediatrician or your family doctor will select the most appropriate formula for your baby. Much of the baby formula sold today is already prepared and sold in a can, ready to feed; some is concentrated and requires the addition of tap water. Both of these forms are far simpler than the "homemade" recipe of evaporated milk, sugar, and water, followed by a sterilization procedure. This traditional procedure is used by less than 10 percent of women who bottle-feed. It is far less expensive but more time-consuming than using a prepared formula. And it is usually not recommended by pediatricians because prepared formulas are modified to meet the nutritional needs of the baby.

If you choose to bottle-feed, and if you will be preparing homemade formula, it is wise to purchase the supplies before your baby is born. Practice the procedure at least once before the baby is born, preferably with some guidance. Be sure to discard the formula after you make it—it will not keep.

Regardless of what is in the bottle, it is reassuring to know that Dad, an older child, or a friend or relative can feed the baby.

*Mary:* "We worked out a system with each of our children. I fed the baby a bottle late at night before I went to sleep. Then Peter would feed the baby if she woke during the night and again before he left for work, while I was still sleeping."

*Peter*: "I had a special time with my daughters, and developed a wonderful closeness with them during those nighttime hours in the easy chair. It wasn't long before the night feedings stopped, but the nighttime routine remained. Throughout the early years, Rachel and Leslie, if they woke, stood in their cribs and called 'Daddy!' "

Your decision to nurse or bottle-feed may depend on your "support staff." Some women feel they need help with housework or other children if they are to be successful with breastfeeding; others choose to bottle-feed and must find dependable help who can be trusted to provide loving care for the baby when mother is away.

*Mary*: "When Rachel was born, Josephine, the woman who cared for me as a child (as well as my brothers and cousins), came to live with us. So our family jumped from two to four. My decision to bottle-feed was supported by Peter, my mother, and Josephine—all of whom thought bottle-feeding was the *only* choice. And most of my friends were choosing to bottle-feed.

"My family and friends, plus my intention to return to work, influenced this decision. Rachel and Leslie both stayed home with Josephine, who offered unbounded love and care. Sometimes each of them came to work, especially if I had a short workday. I was teaching nutrition in a school of nursing at the time, and a car-bed carrier fit nicely by the side of my desk. Mostly, they slept through lectures, meetings, and office hours as both were 'easy' babies, and quick diaper changes and a bottle fit into the plan. Student nurses became more comfortable holding, feeding, and changing babies with Rachel or Leslie in the role of baby."

Many women work because of financial necessity and find that their places of employment have neither policies nor facilities that encourage breastfeeding. It is often easier to choose formula so others can feed the baby, and mother has more flexibility. Baby won't be hungry if mother is delayed.

Working women who decide to breastfeed their babies must

be very dedicated. If at all possible, it is best to wait until the baby is four to six months old before returning to full-time work.

*Anne*: "I did not have a career at that point in my life, though I was working. We decided that having a family was an important part of our 'Grand Plan.' I quit my job to 'manage' the family full-time. I threw myself into parenting the way some people launch their careers. Nursing the baby, morning, noon, night, and a few times in between, was no problem for this earnest mother! It would have been very hard if I had needed to return to work while I was nursing."

If a woman has to return to work, she can express breast milk, either by hand or a mechanical pump, which can then be given to the baby in a bottle. While some women find this works, others experience reduced milk supply as sucking is decreased, and the baby must then be given formula. With the increasing number of working women and the trend toward breastfeeding, we hope that the day will soon come when there are creative day-care facilities that will allow mothers to work away from home and continue to breastfeed.

One mother we know was determined to nurse her baby after she returned to her job as a fashion reporter on the staff of a local newspaper. She said that there were several conditions that made it possible: She had some flexibility in her schedule, allowing for occasional late arrivals and early departures, as well as time midday to express her milk into a bottle for the next day. She had an office where this could be done discreetly. She also had a small refrigerator in her office, where she could store the milk. She nursed her daughter for a year, and said she does not think any of her colleagues even knew she was doing it! This young mother had wanted to stay at home to nurse her baby, but could not do so for financial reasons. Nursing was her way of feeling close to her baby.

Many women want to breastfeed, but like to go out occasionally; they may also be concerned about providing nourishment for their children in case of an emergency that prevents them from being available. There is a difference of opinion about infant formula supplements for breastfed babies. It is true that if a baby is given bottles before he is well established at the breast, he may become confused and refuse one or the other. This happens because two very different sucking techniques are used for the breast and the bottle, and the very young baby cannot master both simultaneously.

A breastfed baby can be introduced to the bottle after about two weeks, and receive one or two bottles a week without interfering with nursing. This is not a problem for the woman who is very confident about nursing, and does not use the bottle as a crutch; the bottle is more likely to interfere when the mother is concerned about "having enough milk," or "being just too nervous to nurse." If bottles are readily available, some women have a tendency to give up quickly when nursing problems develop.

Breastfeeding is practiced in diverse ways in our society. After the first few weeks, some women establish a schedule, and nurse the baby on a fairly regular basis; others continue to nurse on demand, including the baby's needs for comfort or sucking in their nursing regimen. Some women begin weaning to a cup at about six months, while others nurse for two to three years.

At four to five months, the baby who receives formula regularly but is still being nursed may begin to show a definite preference for the bottle. Formula flows much more quickly and with less effort from the bottle, which he may like. A mother must then decide whether to pursue nursing by decreasing the number of bottles, or convert to bottle feeding, or to begin weaning the child and adding solid foods. For the remainder of the first year, formula should be given instead of unmodified cow's milk.[54]

Some women choose to breastfeed for only a few weeks or months to get the baby off to a good start. To breastfeed, even for a short time, is good for the baby.

Because the pendulum of thinking has swung to encouraging breastfeeding as the optimal method of feeding, there is a tendency for women to feel guilty if they choose to bottle-feed. For some there is a concern that they are not "maternal" enough. But babies can be well nourished, both physically and emotionally, on either breast or bottle milk.

## Private Thoughts

Some women may not have considered breastfeeding as a serious option because they think it will affect the shape of their breasts. While nursing does change the breasts temporarily, women who wear well-fitted bras find that their breasts do not sag, and they return to their pre-pregnancy size and shape when the baby is about nine months old. Many women's breasts permanently increase in size as a result of pregnancy, even if the women choose not to breastfeed.

The size and shape of a woman's breasts make little difference to her success in nursing. Nature has determined that every mother, with few exceptions, can nurse her offspring. A woman who has inverted nipples, or who suspects that she has any barrier to breastfeeding, should consult her doctor early in pregnancy about techniques that will prepare her for nursing.

Modesty may be an important deterrent to a woman's decision not to feed her child at the breast. No one says you have to make a production of nursing your baby in public! Many women prefer to nurse privately. Some men are uncomfortable at having their wives nurse their children outside the privacy of home. Also many men are uncomfortable in a room where any woman is nursing. Despite the naturalness of it all, sensitivity is necessary. Riding the bus is usually not the best time for breastfeeding!

If you are "caught," and can't find a comfortable private spot, you can nurse discreetly by adjusting your clothing, or covering your breast with a blanket or diaper. Much of the self-consciousness that women experience when they first begin breastfeeding is lost as they become more comfortable and are assured that what they are doing is very natural and beautiful. There are few situations in which you and your baby cannot find a quiet private place to nurse.

*A real "plus" for the figure-conscious woman who chooses to breastfeed her baby is that the pounds gained during pregnancy are utilized in the production of milk, and most women who choose to breastfeed return to their normal weight more easily than do bottle-feeding mothers.* As the baby nurses, hormones are released that cause the uterus to contract, facilitating its return to normal.

The woman who chooses not to breastfeed usually has as much as 10 pounds of stored fat—Nature's anticipation of breastfeeding, which then doesn't happen. She may need to diet to lose the weight and she can expect to need an injection or medication to cause the uterus to contract.

The discussion up to this point has dealt with the issues that come up when trying to decide how to feed your baby. We will now examine some of the day-to-day practicalities of these two ways of feeding.

## Women Who Breastfeed

There is much to be learned about breastfeeding. There are a number of excellent books and pamphlets available; many are listed in the next chapter. The La Leche League (La Leche means "the milk" in Spanish) provides information and support to breastfeeding women. There may be a La Leche group, or a similar support organization, in your area which will meet your needs and interests.

Belonging to a support group is not essential for successful breastfeeding, but having some source of information and encouragement is one of the most critical factors. *Breastfeeding does not come naturally; it has to be learned.*

Dr. Dana Raphael, an anthropologist, noted that in cultures where women breastfeed their babies, a system of training and support exists. A *doula*, or helper, assists the new mother and teaches her the art of mothering.[38] The duola may help with the household chores, the other children, etc., but her primary task is to teach the new mother the tricks of caring for and feeding her baby.

*Anne*: "My doula was a book by Niles Newton called *The Family Book of Child Care*.[32] I think at that time in my life I looked more to books than to other people for advice. Dr. Newton not only convinced me that breastfeeding was best, but she told me how to do it. I remember one time when my nipple cracked and started to bleed; I was horrified, and afraid to nurse the baby. What a comfort to find advice in the book that told me just what to do! Twenty years is a long time to wait to say thank you—'Thank you, Niles Newton!'"

In our society, your doula may be a friend or relative who

can provide practical tips on breastfeeding and child care and give encouragement during the first weeks. The La Leche League is the best known breastfeeding support group. They offer information and support through local groups. You may or may not be comfortable with group situations: the members, the leadership, or the philosophy, which tends to be unrestricted breastfeeding. If it is not right for you, call the public relations department of your local hospital or talk with someone on their pediatrics or OB/GYN staff about other support groups in your area. If you tried unsuccessfully to breastfeed a child before, a doula may be just what you need. Find yourself a doula before your baby is born!

If you decide to breastfeed your baby, you will want a physician who is supportive during your pregnancy. You might ask, when you are in the process of choosing a doctor, how many of his or her patients breastfeed, whether breastfeeding preparation is included in the doctor's prenatal care, and whether you can have an opportunity to nurse your baby immediately after delivery and on demand during your hospital stay. Because babies nurse better if their mothers have not been heavily sedated during delivery, you should ask your doctor about the type of anesthetic to be used during delivery. While your doctor may give you medication for pain, drugs that interfere with the initiation of breastfeeding can generally be avoided. Make sure the attending physician during delivery knows that you intend to breastfeed, so you will not be given medication to stop your milk from coming in.

Women who require Cesarean deliveries can successfully breastfeed soon after the baby is born. It helps ease the disappointment that some women feel when they are unable to deliver vaginally as planned, especially if they have prepared for a natural childbirth delivery. Discuss this possibility so you will know the degree to which the doctor will cooperate with your commitment to breastfeed.

## Producing Grade A Milk

Many women are distressed when they see that the substance coming from their breast is a yellowish transparent liquid that does not look at all like milk. This substance, which precedes regular milk, is *colostrum*. The nursing baby receives colostrum during the first three to five days of life, until the milk comes in. Some women may find that the colostrum does not flow immediately, but only after the baby sucks at her breast. This is quite normal, and should not cause her to worry; even a little will meet the baby's needs.

Hand-expressing a few drops of colostrum in the last months of pregnancy has been commonly recommended. The most current thinking, however, is that there may be some disadvantages to expressing colostrum during pregnancy.[16]

* It opens up ducts to possible infection.
* It should be "saved" for the baby (there is no evidence to indicate whether there is a fixed amount or if more is produced to make up for what has been expressed).
* Hand-expressing may trigger contractions and premature labor.

"If we could, we'd welcome every baby into the world with a colostrum cocktail," said Dr. Mary Ann Neifert, of the University of Colorado.[173] A single feeding of colostrum may increase his immunity to infections during the first six months of his life, or longer, and protect him from allergic reactions well into his second year.[37]

Colostrum contains more protein, less sugar, and much less fat than mature milk. It aids in the establishment of the proper "healthy" bacteria and acidity in the baby's digestive tract, which provides protection against gastrointestinal infections.

Colostrum changes to transitional milk between the third and sixth day, and by about the tenth day most changes have occurred. The milk supply is not stable in composition and quantity until the end of the first month.

### Quality and Quantity

Mother Nature has a will for babies to survive and produces some breast milk even when women have poor diets.

Harriet Danzyger, R.D., Clinical Dietitian at Northwestern Memorial Hospital, Prentice Women's Hospital and Maternity Center, said, "There is a real question as to the amount of milk produced by women whose diets are poor. Recent evidence suggests that less milk is produced. Women I counsel report that when they reduce their caloric intake or skip meals, their breast milk production is substantially decreased."

The major components of milk can be drawn from the mother's reserves. Vitamins, and to a lesser extent minerals, which are important for optimal health, depend more on the mother's diet. The mother who neglects her diet when she is breastfeeding jeopardizes her own health and her baby's. She needs to replenish the reserves that are used for the milk and provide nutrients that will help her maintain the stamina and sense of well-being that are necessary if she is to successfully breastfeed her child. R. G. Whitehead, in a 1979 issue of the *Postgraduate Medical Journal*, said it well: *"Breast milk is not a gift: the nutrients contained in milk do not materialize out of thin air. Either directly or indirectly they must come from the mother's diet."*[143]

## Breastfeeding and Your Diet

### Calories

Those extra pounds you gained during pregnancy are insurance that calories will be available for milk. If you gained within the normal range, the fat reserves (approximately 8 pounds) will be depleted by breastfeeding in about three months.

It takes about 500 calories each day, in addition to those drawn from fat stores, to make an adequate supply of milk. For this reason, the RDAs during lactation recommend an increase of 500 calories in your diet. These calories are very efficiently used and should not result in your gaining additional weight.

Many women are anxious to shed the extra pounds of pregnancy immediately after delivery. It is important not to go on a crash diet, however, or you may find yourself fatigued and unable to produce enough milk to nourish your baby. Your baby does not need a "second-hand" weight reduction diet during a period of rapid growth!

*Implications for Food Choices* If you are not losing weight as quickly as you would like, take another look at your daily diet. Continue to eat the nutritious foods but find sources of sugar and fat that can be eliminated. Instead of eating extra calories for fuel—*burn your stored fat as fuel!*

### Protein

Most human milk is adequate in protein to meet the needs for the baby's growth until he is about six months old. Protein for milk takes precedence over protein to meet the mother's needs, so it is important that you consume extra protein during lactation to prevent your body stores from becoming depleted.

There is no specific place in our body to store protein for emergency use. So when protein is withdrawn from "stores" it means that your muscles and vital organs lose part of their structural protein.

*Implications for Food Choices* While women need less protein during lactation than during pregnancy, the RDAs suggest 20 grams of protein in excess of pre-pregnancy need. You need an extra 30 grams of protein in pregnancy, so if you continue your pregnancy diet, you have plenty of protein.

### Fat

There are no recommendations for fat intake during lactation, but the amount of saturated or polyunsaturated fat the nursing mother consumes is reflected in the fat composition in her milk. Polyunsaturated dietary fat is a source of essential fatty acids, which pass through to the baby.

### Vitamins

The breastfed baby depends on the mother's diet to provide water-soluble vitamins, especially vitamins C, $B_6$, thiamin, and riboflavin. The human lactation system processes the fragile water-soluble vitamins so that maximum amounts are passed to the nursing baby.

The fat-soluble vitamins (A, D, E, and K) do not pass as easily from the mother's bloodstream into breast milk. The vitamin A in mother's milk is strongly influenced by her diet.[50] The vitamin D in human milk has recently been found in a water-soluble form, but researchers do not know whether it is utilized. Many doctors prescribe vitamin D supplements for breastfed babies. Mother's milk contains some vitamin K after the fourth day of nursing, but newborns are routinely given this vitamin to protect them from hemorrhaging.

*Implications for Food Choices* The vitamins needed in larger amounts during lactation than during pregnancy include significant increases in vitamins A, C, and niacin, and modest increases in vitamins E, thiamin, and riboflavin. The nutrient with the biggest increase is vitamin C; this need can be easily met with the selection of two good vitamin C sources each day from the list provided in Chapter 7.

## Minerals

■ *Iron* The amount of iron in breast milk is low, and it is not affected by the mother's diet. However, mothers with adequate iron intakes during pregnancy usually give birth to babies that have enough iron stored in their livers to last for four to six months when milk is the sole diet. If the mother did not have adequate iron during pregnancy to allow the baby's reserves to grow, he will be deficient after birth. Because of the prevalence of inadequate iron reserves, many physicians prescribe supplementary iron to both the mother and baby for three to four months after birth. The NRC recommends that iron supplements be continued after delivery. Since menstruation is delayed by breastfeeding, the mother conserves her iron stores after the baby is born. During breastfeeding, the mother needs adequate iron to meet her own needs and to replace blood lost during delivery.

■ *Calcium* The calcium level of human milk is relatively constant regardless of the mother's diet.[80] But the mother who is calcium-deficient risks having the calcium in her bones used to maintain the levels in her milk. This weakens her bone strength and may make her more susceptible to bone fractures later in life. The milk, yogurt, or other calcium-rich foods you've learned to love during pregnancy should continue to play a prominent role in your diet during lactation.

■ *Fluoride* Studies are under way to determine whether mothers who drink fluoridated water pass enough through in their milk to meet their baby's needs. In 1979, the American Academy of Pediatrics determined that all breastfed babies should receive .25 milligram supplementary fluoride, regardless of their mother's intake. A nursing mother should continue to follow the advice given on fluoride in Chapter 6 to meet her own needs.

## Liquids

There is no evidence that drinking more water, or any other fluid or food, causes a direct increase in the amount of milk produced.[80] However, when any fluid leaves the body, it draws on the bloodstream and body cells to release water. Thus, the production of milk creates a need for more fluids to avoid dehydration. Thirst is the body's signal to replace liquid.

*Implications for Food Choices* The easiest and most satisfactory way to meet the need for liquids is to increase the consumption of milk and fruit juices, which together meet the needs for extra calcium and vitamin C. The remainder of the fluid need can be met by a few glasses of "no-cal" water. Soups and moderate amounts of coffee, tea, or lemonade also contribute to fluid needs, but large amounts of caffeine-containing beverages should be avoided because caffeine can pass from your bloodstream into milk and make the baby fretful.[85]

Many women have heard that drinking beer increases milk production. It is not clear whether this belief is physiological, psychological, or an "old wives' tale." Perhaps it is a bit of each. Beer does provide fluid and its alcohol causes some women to relax. But it is *not* a nutritious beverage. It contains a bit of brewer's yeast, which has some B vitamins, particularly niacin, but the total of nutrients does not make a significant contribution to your diet. The effect of alcohol is clearly negative as it passes from the mother's bloodstream into her milk. Large amounts of alcohol are bad for both you and baby, but there is no evidence that a can or two of beer causes harm. If you are drinking beer for the brewer's yeast, consider taking the brewer's yeast without its alcohol companion. A varied diet does not require supplementation with brewer's yeast. Again, ask your doctor.

## Vegetarian Nursing Mothers

A sensible vegetarian diet that includes sufficient calories and protein is adequate for both mother and baby during lactation. The mother needs to pay special attention to meeting the needs for calcium, riboflavin, and thiamin. If she eats no animal products, she may need a $B_{12}$ supplement to prevent anemia in both herself and her baby. If she does not drink milk, the calcium sources she used during pregnancy should be continued.

Vegetarian mothers should be encouraged to consume their extra calories from foods that are sources of high-quality protein obtained from complementary grains, nuts, vegetables, legumes, and dairy products.

## Recommended Nutrients for Lactation

Successful lactation can be achieved at various levels of nutrient intake. If care is taken to choose a varied and balanced diet, both Mom and baby will benefit. Lactation can be an enormous drain on the mother; she must take care to maintain her health. The RDAs reflect a margin for safety for this purpose and are sufficient to provide nutrients to the baby that can be given through breast milk. The RDAs for lactation are included in the chart on page 44.

### Dietary Supplements During Lactation

Many lactating women are advised to continue taking pre-natal vitamin-mineral supplements during the first few months of breastfeeding. L. J. Filer, Jr., a prominent researcher at the University of Iowa College of Medicine, contends that "in-creased needs can be provided by a well-balanced diet. Thus, nutritional supplements are generally unnecessary except when there is a deficient intake of one or more nutrients."[80]

Dr. Filer does, however, recommend supplemental iron to replenish stores lost in pregnancy for all postpartum women, whether they breast- or bottle-feed their infants.

Since there are differences in medical opinion as well as individual differences among women, you should ask your obstetrician or pediatrician about vitamin-mineral supplementation when you are breastfeeding.

## Contaminants in Breast Milk

Breast milk is not always 100 percent "pure." The composition of the milk reflects the environment and the mother's personal habits which, in some cases, may not be the best habits for growing babies.

We discussed the effects of caffeine and alcohol earlier in this chapter. The conscientious mother wants to know about *any* substance that is potentially harmful to the baby.

### Nicotine

We hope that you have stopped or cut down on smoking during pregnancy. We hope you can keep from smoking or at least will be moderate in your use of cigarettes during lactation. Smoking has been shown in both humans and experimental animals to reduce the amount of milk produced.[39] There is no proof that smoking while you nurse endangers the baby; however, since nicotine is a toxic substance, it cannot be recommended.

### Marijuana

The most active ingredient in marijuana is fat-soluble, and therefore passes along in breast milk. Long-term effects are not yet known, but it is known that marijuana contains a chemical that disrupts the production of hormones in both the mother and child.[39]

### Drugs

Before you take *any* drug, prescription or over-the-counter, be sure to find out if it is passed through breast milk and poses a threat to the nursing infant. The infant's kidneys and liver may be unable to excrete or detoxify these drugs. If you choose to breastfeed, ask your doctor for a list of permitted over-the-counter drugs, and take no prescription drugs without specific advice that they are safe for your baby. Many common drugs, such as aspirin, Valium, and a variety of antibiotics, can be dangerous to your baby. Your taking large amounts of aspirin, which is usually assumed to be quite safe, can cause your newborn baby to hemorrhage.[136]

Some women have been advised to wean if they require medications, but this does not take into account the mother's feelings about weaning, what the baby experiences if suddenly taken from the breast, or the loss to the baby of the positive factors in the mother's milk. Ask your physician if there is another way to treat the illness, or if simply waiting it out with no medication is a real threat to your health.

Many drugs have little or no effect on the nursing infant because they do not pass through into milk. Have your doctor check a current reference that tells potential danger of drugs to breastfeeding, and prescribe the one with the least risks.[142] The effects of some drugs may appear to be very minimal, but trace amounts absorbed by the baby can lead to an allergic reaction to that drug at a later time.[85]

Take prescribed medications at the beginning of nursing (it will not have time to pass into the milk) or just after nursing (so levels will be reduced before the next nursing).

## Oral Contraceptives

There have been a number of studies that demonstrate that traditional oral contraceptives that contain both estrogen and progestin reduce the quantity and quality of breast milk. The newer progestin-only type (low-dosage or mini-pills) are preferable during lactation as they do not seem to limit milk production and impair the infant's growth.[56] The evidence is not yet in on the long-term effects.

Although it is known that lactation was a primitive form of birth control, it is not a reliable method of planned parenthood. Methods of contraception during lactation should be discussed with your obstetrician or family physician.

## Food Additives, Artificial Sweeteners

Very little is known about specific food additives or artificial sweeteners and their potential for transmittal through breast milk. Cyclamate, an artificial sweetener banned in the United States but sold in Canada, has been studied as a component of diet drinks. Four cans were consumed each day for a week. After one week, some milk was expressed and evaluated for cyclamates. Small amounts were found in the milk, but far fewer than the concentration in the mother's bloodstream.[167]

Aspartame is an artificial sweetener recently approved by the Food and Drug Administration for use in the United States. We do not yet know about its effects in pregnancy and lactation. Every food containing aspartame will be labeled, making identification easier for pregnant and lactating women.

## PCBs, DDT and Other Environmental Contaminants

There has been a great deal of concern about environmental contaminants in breast milk. Over the last half-century, chemicals have been employed in a variety of industrial uses and have been polluting the environment. The public was alarmed to discover increased incidences of cancer and birth defects in exposed populations, and high levels of contaminants in the breast milk of these women.

With the awareness of the health hazard posed by contaminants, their use in North America has been greatly reduced in recent years. High levels of DDT and related compounds have been found in the breast milk of some women in Guatemala and Finland,[39] and PCBs were found in some contaminated pregnant Japanese women.[29] But in our search of the literature, we were unable to find documentation of dangerously high levels of PCBs (polychlorinated biphenyls) or DDT in the diets of American women except in cases where the women regularly worked with or ate fish caught by sportfishing in contaminated waters.

If there is a question about breast milk contamination, ask your state health department to measure for levels of those compounds. Doctors generally agree that the benefits of breast-feeding greatly outweigh the risks of environmental contaminants except for individual women exposed to high levels of a specific contaminant.

There are several things you can do to minimize the

potential of adding contaminants to your diet:

* Wash fruits and vegetables thoroughly.
* Since PCBs are found in fat, decrease fat in your diet.
* Pregnant and lactating women should not eat fish from lakes and rivers that have been contaminated by PCBs.
* Pregnant and lactating women should avoid exposure to industrial chemicals, pesticides, and "carbon" paper that contains no carbons.[163]

## Foods That Cause Gas

There is no evidence that specific foods cause the baby to become upset, but a food that causes *you* discomfort may very well create a similar effect in your baby. Large quantities of such strongly flavored foods as onions, cabbage, garlic, or beans have been reported to cause fussiness in a breastfed infant. Coffee and cocoa contain stimulants that some babies cannot tolerate. Watch for a pattern of baby discomfort and see if it relates to consumption of a specific food. If you find a correlation exists, it is simple enough to avoid the food while you are nursing.

This section is not a complete guide to breastfeeding. It is intended to give you enough information about the process to help you decide whether or not you want to breastfeed your baby. Specific information on how to breastfeed is available from the resources listed in Chapter 11, from your physician, or from a breastfeeding support group.

## The Bottle-Fed Baby

We have already said enough about infant formulas for you to realize that they are not all the same. There is no way of knowing exactly which will be best for your baby. While you are in the hospital, the doctor (usually the pediatrician) will order a specific formula based on the needs of your baby including weight, family history of allergies, and other factors. The baby will be observed to be sure that the formula is well tolerated. The real test will be whether your child does well on it during his first weeks and months. If there are problems, another formula will be substituted.

## A MENU FOR NEWBORNS [157]

| Optimal choice | Breast milk | |
| --- | --- | --- |
| Good | Commercial formulas | Many good ones are available, including a number of special-purpose formulas. Most have vitamins and minerals added so supplements are not necessary. |
| Acceptable Only if Supplemented (Not Usually Recommended) | Formula made from evaporated whole cow's milk | Lacks vitamins C and E. Requires supplementary vitamins to be given. The evaporation process reduces the size of the protein acid and improves digestibility. Must be diluted with water and have sugar added. |
| Not Acceptable Until One Year[121] | Fresh whole cow's milk | Cow's-milk protein, if unaltered by processing, is hard for baby to digest. The butterfat is poorly utilized. Research shows that fresh milk can cause gastrointestinal bleeding, leading to anemia in young infants. |
| Not Acceptable | 2% milk, skim milk | Does not provide adequate fat or essential fatty acids. Fat is necessary early in life for brain and nervous-system development. These forms of milk should not be used during the first eighteen months of life. |

Most liquid formulas contain about twenty calories per ounce, but some have more calories per ounce for low-birthweight babies. Formulas differ in sources of protein, fat, and carbohydrate. There are many formulas available. In our area, the most popular ones are Isomil, Enfamil, and Similac.

*Most popular commercial formulas come in a concentrated form to which tap or boiled water must be added, or as a ready-to-serve liquid that can be poured directly into a clean bottle.* Bottles can be prepared singly or for a whole day. They must be refrigerated once they are prepared.

It is not necessary to sterilize or even to warm formulas as long as the baby likes what he gets. Babies used to room-temperature formula like it that way; babies used to chilled

## NUTRIENT SOURCES IN COMMERCIAL INFANT FORMULAS

|  | Protein | Fat | Carbohydrate |
|---|---|---|---|
| Isomil | soy isolate | soy and coconut oils | corn syrup and sucrose |
| Enfamil, Similac (with or without iron) | cow's milk | soy and coconut oils | lactose |

Other formulas use meat, casein, or whey as the protein; some use corn, safflower, or sesame oil as the fat; some use tapioca, maltose, or dextrose as the carbohydrate.

formulas like it at that temperature. If it makes *you* feel better to give your baby a warm bottle, and the baby is happy with it, then do so. You can warm it up by running it under hot water for a minute or two.

The most important aspect of formula preparation is *sanitation*. The bottles and nipples must be absolutely clean. The formula in an opened can may be kept, refrigerated, for no more than twenty-four hours. Milk left from one feeding should not be saved for another feeding, no matter how wasteful that may seem. Bacteria from the baby's mouth contaminates the formula and can cause illness if it is saved and offered at the next meal.

There are two aspects that come automatically with breast-feeding that can also be practiced when you bottle-feed your baby.

1. *Do not overfeed the baby.* Do not try to make the baby empty the bottle. This practice fosters eating past satisfaction and increases the possibility of weight-control problems throughout life. Breastfed babies decide when to stop sucking, and that's that. If your baby refuses to take any more of his bottle, he may be full—let him be the judge. If this happens consistently, pour less formula in the bottles.

2. *Hold and cuddle the baby at feeding time.* Being held gives your baby a sense of security that does not come from a

propped bottle. If baby vomits or chokes, you will be there to help. Let Dad or other members of the family share the joy of holding and cuddling the baby while baby is being fed.

## Breast or Bottle? A Summary

### Reasons for Breastfeeding

* Breast milk is the nutritionally superior food for human babies.
* Breast milk is easily absorbed and digested by infants. Few upsets, constipation, diarrhea, and allergies occur.
* Babies who are breastfed are protected against illness by special disease-fighting antibodies in the milk.
* The action of sucking promotes good tooth, jaw, and palate formation.
* Nursing utilizes the mother's fat reserves to make milk, helps control post-delivery bleeding, and encourages the return of the uterus to normal without the use of medication.
* Breast milk is always ready for the baby—sterile and fresh.
* Nursing promotes bonding between the mother and baby.
* Breastfeeding helps control the tendency of babies to be overfed because there is no bottle to empty.
* Breastfeeding, even with the addition of foods to the mother's diet, is less expensive than formula.
* Breastfeeding eliminates the need for bottles, bottle washing, and carrying bottles around.

### Reasons for Bottle-Feeding

* Some women may find the idea of nursing distasteful.
* Nursing may not be accepted by the mother's mate or by others whose support she values.
* The mother's lifestyle may not allow her to give the time

required to nurse, especially if she returns to work shortly after the baby's birth.

* A woman may have had a previous unpleasant experience with nursing.
* The father, older children, and others can share in the care of the infant.
* The mother can be more independent.
* A woman who is uneasy about caring for a newborn, can have an exact measure of her baby's food intake.
* Some women may have physical problems that prevent them from nursing. For instance, women who must receive certain medications may be advised not to breast-feed.
* There are many special-purpose formulas available for babies with particular needs.

We know you are as concerned about getting your baby off to a good start as you were about providing optimal care during pregnancy. There is no question about the method that is preferred by health professionals, but if breastfeeding isn't right for you, then it isn't better for your child. *Good parenting is a great deal more important than the kind of milk you give your baby.*

# 11.
# Remarks, Resources and References

Rather than just "letting it happen" or passively waiting for medical professionals to tell them what to do, women today are participating in the management of pregnancy. We hope that this book has helped you understand the role of nutrition during pregnancy.

There may be some aspects you want to know more about, or you may have special needs that are beyond the scope of this book. A number of excellent resources are available.

In addition to printed materials, you may want to seek out individuals or groups that provide support and understanding to help you make decisions affecting your pregnancy and your baby's health.

## Finding Local Resources

Information about special circumstances related to pregnancy is available from hospitals, local health organizations, individual counselors, and support groups. Support groups are often started by women who have experienced a particular situation, and feel that other women who have the same problem can benefit from sharing with one another. Support groups exist for mothers of twins, for diabetic mothers, for breastfeeding mothers, for single mothers, for first-time mothers, and so on.

Community resources are sometimes difficult to track down. It may take several calls.

1. Ask your doctor or nurse.
2. Call the largest (or best) hospital nearest you and ask for information from:

   * the Nursing Department;
   * the Public Relations Department;
   * the Obstetrics Department.

   In Chicago, Northwestern Memorial Hospital has an excellent resource center that is open to the public. There is information about many health topics, including pregnancy, which has been reviewed by medical professionals. There may be a hospital in your area that has a similar facility.
3. Call your local Department of Public Health and talk with the public health nutritionist.
4. Enter into conversation with women in your doctor's waiting room.
5. Call a local hospital and ask to talk with a registered dietitian who can tell you how to contact the Dietetic Association in your state. Many state associations have lists of registered dietitians who do individual nutrition counseling.
6. Write or call the health editor or writer of the nearest metropolitan or neighborhood newspaper. He or she is likely to know about programs and services available to the public.

## National Resources

The American College of Obstetricians and Gynecologists
Resource Center
600 Maryland Avenue, S.W., Suite 300E
Washington, DC 20024-2588

> ACOG has published a Patient Information Booklet Series covering many topics.

The Center for the Study of Multiple Gestation
Suite 463-5
333 East Superior Street
Chicago, IL 60601

> Expecting twins, triplets, more? If so, contact the center for a listing of information, support groups, and available services.

La Leche League International
9616 Minneapolis Avenue
Franklin Park, IL 60131

> This organization offers help and support for nursing mothers. Send for a catalog of available materials and local affiliates.

Maternity Center Association
48 East 92 Street
New York, NY 10028

> Providers of booklets and materials on topics related to pregnancy.

March of Dimes Birth Defects Foundation
1275 Mamaroneck Avenue
White Plains, NY 10605

> The March of Dimes objectives include the prevention of birth defects and improving the outcome of pregnancy. There are local chapters throughout the country that provide public health education and community services. They publish a number of excellent books, pamphlets, films, and other materials.

Society for Nutrition Education
1736 Franklin Street
Oakland, CA 94612

> SNE has produced a wonderful film, called "Great Expectations," about nutrition and pregnancy. The film is available in English and Spanish. It is available from many sources, including your

local chapter of the March of Dimes. SNE also has a fifteen-page bibliography, titled "Pregnancy and Nutrition," available for $3.00.

Women, Infants, Children Program (WIC)
U.S. Department of Agriculture
Food and Nutrition Service
Washington, DC 20250

If your income is low, you may be eligible for supplemental food during pregnancy and breastfeeding and for your infant. There is no central directory of services. To find the nearest program, call your local Department of Health.

## Selected Books by Topic

To be included on the following list, books had to meet 2 criteria:
1. *Books have been reviewed and approved for content* by the medical, nursing, or nutrition staff of Northwestern Memorial Hospital in Chicago.
2. Each book has been recommended by the Coordinator of the Northwestern Memorial Hospital Health Resource Center because *it is popular and enjoyed by the general public.*

These resources are available in libraries or bookstores. They are excellent sources of information in areas related to nutrition in pregnancy that are not within the scope of this book.

We have not included cookbooks because there are many wonderful cookbooks and your favorite one surely has recipes that are both healthful and delicious.

### General Pregnancy

Tracy Hotchner. *Pregnancy and Childbirth: The Complete Guide for a New Life.* (New York: Avon, 1979).

Boston Children's Medical Center. *Pregnancy, Birth and the Newborn Baby.* (New York: Delacorte Press, 1972).

Lennart Nilsson and A. Ingelman-Sundberg. *A Child Is Born: The Drama of Life Before Birth.* (New York: Dell Publishing, 1980).

Clark Gillespie. *Your Pregnancy, Month by Month.* (New York: Harper & Row, 1977).

### Pregnancy at Various Ages

Linda Barr and Catherine Monserrat. *Teenage Pregnancy: A New Beginning.* (Albuquerque: New Futures, 1978).

Daniel Jay Baum. *Teenage Pregnancy.* (New York: Beaufort Books, 1980).

Howard R. Lewis and Martha A. Lewis. *The Parents' Guide to Teenage Sex and Pregnancy.* (New York: St. Martin's Press, 1980).

Elizabeth Bing and Libby Coleman. *Having a Baby After 30.* (New York: Bantam, 1980).

Jane Price. *You're Not Too Old to Have a Baby.* (New York: Farrar, Straus, Giroux, 1977).

Sylvia P. Rubin. *It's Not Too Late to Have a Baby.* (Englewood Cliffs, NJ: Prentice-Hall, 1980).

## Multiple Births

Elizabeth Noble. *Having Twins.* (Boston: Houghton Mifflin, 1980).

*Breastfeeding Your Twins.* To order, send $1.00 to:
    The Center for the Study of Multiple Gestation
    Suite 463-5
    333 East Superior Street
    Chicago, IL 60601

## Fathering

Sam Bittman and Sue Rosenberg Zalk. *Expectant Fathers.* (New York: Ballantine, 1978).

Peter Mayle. *How to Be a Pregnant Father.* (Secaucus, NJ: Lyle Stuart, 1979).

## Exercise and Fitness

Elizabeth Bing. *Moving Through Pregnancy.* (New York: Bantam, 1975).

Elizabeth Noble. *Essential Exercises for the Childbearing Years.* (Boston: Houghton Mifflin, 1976).

## Vegetarianism

Frances Moore Lappé. *Diet for a Small Planet,* Revised Edition. (New York: Ballantine, 1975).

Laurel Robertson, Carol Flinders, and Bronwen Godfrey. *Laurel's Kitchen.* (Berkeley, CA: Nilgiri Press, 1976).

Victor Zurbel. *The Vegetarian Family* (Englewood Cliffs, NJ: Prentice-Hall, 1978).

### Breastfeeding

Marvin S. Eiger and Sally W. Olds. *The Complete Book of Breastfeeding.* (New York: Workman Publishing, 1976).

Karen Pryor. *Nursing Your Baby.* (New York: Harper & Row, 1973).

Dana Raphael. *The Tender Gift: Breastfeeding.* (New York: Schocken, 1976).

## Our Special Resources

There were many people who provided "essential nutrients" that went into the making of this book.

We acknowledge the support and encouragement, as well as the technical expertise, we received from the consulting authorities listed at the front of the book, as well as from the numerous health professionals who shared our goal of helping women have good pregnancies and healthy babies.

We appreciate the assistance of Carole Chambers, Ph.D., in the development of the manuscript, and Christine Washington and Chester Height for their efforts in preparing the manuscript. We thank the staff of McGraw-Hill and our devoted agent, Jane Jordan Browne, especially for their support and encouragement during the final labor.

Keith Taylor, who illustrated the book, had no previous experience with pregnancy. He read the chapters before he drew the pictures. His drawings were clear evidence that he understood what we were saying.

Our families, husbands, children, and friends were asked to share their lives with you in these pages. They provided nourishment and encouraged us throughout the nine months that we researched and wrote this book.

We have delivered. The baby's name: *Pickles and Ice Cream!*

## Answers to Quick Quizzes

### Chapter 2

| | | | |
|---|---|---|---|
| 1. False | | 6. True |
| 2. True | | 7. True |
| 3. True | | 8. True |
| 4. False | | 9. False |
| 5. True | | 10. False |

### Chapter 4

| | | | |
|---|---|---|---|
| 1. False | | 6. True |
| 2. False | | 7. False |
| 3. False | | 8. True |
| 4. True | | 9. True |
| 5. False | | 10. True |

### Chapter 5

| | | | |
|---|---|---|---|
| 1. D | | 6. False |
| 2. C | | 7. False |
| 3. D | | 8. True |
| 4. A | | 9. True |
| 5. B | | 10. False |

### Chapter 6

| | | | |
|---|---|---|---|
| 1. Vitamin D | | 6. True |
| 2. Iodine | | 7. False |
| 3. Milk or Cheese | | 8. True |
| 4. Fluorine | | 9. False |
| 5. Iron | | 10. False |

### Chapter 8

| | | | |
|---|---|---|---|
| 1. False | | 6. False |
| 2. False | | 7. True |
| 3. True | | 8. True |
| 4. True | | 9. False |
| 5. False | | 10. False |

# Bibliography

**Books**

1. Anderson, Garland D. "Clinical Implications of Recent Basic Research in Prenatal Patients." In *Nutrition in Pregnancy*, edited by Emery A. Wilson. Lexington: University of Kentucky, 1980.

2. Annis, Linda F. *The Child Before Birth*. Ithaca, NY: Cornell University Press, 1978.

3. Boston Women's Health Book Collective. *Our Bodies, Ourselves*. New York: Simon & Schuster, 1973.

4. Brody, Jane E. *Jane Brody's Nutrition Book*. New York: W. W. Norton, 1981.

5. Chesley, L. "False Steps in the Study of Pre-eclampsia." In *Hypertension and Pregnancy*, edited by M. D. Lindheimer, A. I. Katz, and F. P. Zuspan. New York: Wylie Medical, 1976.

6. Committee on Dietary Allowances. *Recommended Dietary Allowances*. 9th ed. Washington, D.C.: National Academy of Sciences, 1980.

7. Consumer Reports. *The Medicine Show*. New York: The Consumer Union, 1974.

8. Cornacchia, Harold J., and Barrett, Stephen. *Consumer Health: A Guide to Intelligent Decisions*. 2nd ed. St. Louis: C. V. Mosby, 1980.

9. Coustan, Donald R., and Garvey, Sheila. *The Baby Team: A Positive Approach to Pregnancy with Diabetes*. St. Louis: Monoject—Division of Sherwood Medical, 1979.

10. Creamer, Effie. "The Pregnant Diabetic—A Nutritionist's View." In *Nutrition in Pregnancy*, edited by Emery A. Wilson. Lexington: University of Kentucky, 1980.

11. Duhring, John L. "The Pregnant Diabetic: An Obstetrician's View." In *Nutrition in Pregnancy*, edited by Emery A. Wilson. Lexington: University of Kentucky, 1980.

12. Eiger, Marvin S., and Olds, Sally Wendkos. *The Complete Book of Breastfeeding*. New York: Workman Publishing, 1972.

13. Ewy, Donna, and Ewy, Roger. *Preparation for Breastfeeding*. New York: Doubleday, 1975.

14. Filer, Lloyd J., Jr. "Relationship of Nutrition to Lactation and Newborn Development." In *Nutritional Impact on Women*, edited by K. S. Moglissi and T. N. Evans. New York: Harper & Row, 1977.

15. Foman, S. *Infant Nutrition*. 2nd. ed. Philadelphia: W. B. Saunders, 1974.

16. Goldfarb, Johanna, and Tibbetts, Edith. *Breastfeeding Handbook: A Practical Reference for Physicians, Nurses, and Other Health Professionals*. Hillside, NJ: Enslow Publishers, 1980.

17. Gots, Ronald E., and Gots, Barbara A. *Caring for Your Unborn Child*. New York: Bantam Books, 1977.

18. Guthrie, Helen Andrews. *Introductory Nutrition*. 3rd ed. St. Louis: C. V. Mosby, 1975.

19. Hamilton, Eva May N., and Whitney, Eleanor N. *Nutrition: Concepts and Controversies*. St. Paul: West Publishing, 1979.

20. Herbert, Victor. *Nutrition Cultism: Facts and Fictions*. Philadelphia: George F. Stickley, 1980.

21. Hurley, Lucille S. *Developmental Nutrition*. Englewood Cliffs, NJ: Prentice-Hall, 1980.

22. Jackson, George W. "Substance Abuse/Addiction: Effects on Pregnancy." In *Nutrition in Pregnancy*, edited by Emery A. Wilson. Lexington: University of Kentucky, 1980.

23. Jacobson, Howard N. "Weight and Weight Gain in Pregnancy." In *Clinics in Perinatology*, edited by L. A. Barness and R. M. Pitkin. Philadelphia: W. B. Saunders, 1975.

24. Judges 13:4, 13:7.

25. Kreutler, Patricia A. *Nutrition in Perspective*. Englewood Cliffs, NJ: Prentice-Hall, 1980.

26. La Leche League International. *The Womanly Art of Breastfeeding*. Franklin Park, IL: La Leche League, 1958.

27. Lambert-Lagacé, Louise. *Feeding Your Child*. Cambridge, Ontario: Habitex Books, Collier-Macmillan Canada, 1976.

28. Lavery, J. Patrick. "Hypertensive Disorders of Pregnancy." In *Nutrition in Pregnancy*, edited by Emery A. Wilson. Lexington: University of Kentucky, 1980.

29. Lawrence, R. *Breast-feeding: A Guide for the Medical Profession*. St. Louis: C. V. Mosby, 1980.

30. Lerch, Constance, and Bliss, Virginia. *Maternity Nursing*. 3rd ed. St. Louis: C. V. Mosby, 1978.

31. Middleton, Katherine, and Hess, Mary Abbott. *The Art of Cooking for the Diabetic*. Chicago: Contemporary Books, 1978.

32. Newton, Niles. *The Family Book of Child Care*. New York: Harper & Bros., 1957.

33. Ouellette, Eileen M., and Rosett, Henry L. "The Effect of Maternal Alcohol Ingestion During Pregnancy on Offspring." In *Nutritional Impact on Women*, edited by K. S. Moglissi and T. N. Evans. New York: Harper & Row, 1977.

34. Pennington, Jean A. T., and Church, Helen Nichols. *Food Values of Portions Commonly Used*. 13th ed. New York: Harper & Row, 1980.

35. Pitkin, Roy M. In *Risks in the Practice of Modern Obstetrics*, edited by S. Aladjem. 2nd ed. St. Louis: C. V. Mosby, 1975.

36. Pitkin, Roy M. In *Nutritional Support of Medical Practice*, edited by C. E. Anderson, D. B. Coursin, and H. A. Schneider. New York: Harper & Row, 1977.

37. Pryor, Karen. *Nursing Your Baby*. New York: Harper & Row, 1973.

38. Raphael, Dana. *The Tender Gift: Breast Feeding*. New York: Schocken Books, 1976.

39. Ray, Oakley. *Drugs, Society and Human Behavior*. 2nd ed. St. Louis: C. V. Mosby, 1978.

40. Shier, Robert W. "Changes in Blood Volume During Pregnancy." In *Nutrition in Pregnancy*, edited by Emery A. Wilson. Lexington: University of Kentucky, 1980.

41. Timiras, P. S. *Developmental Physiology and Aging*. New York: Macmillan, 1972.

42. Tinklenberg, J. R., ed. *Marijuana and Health Hazards: Methodological Issues in Current Research*. New York: Academic Press, 1975.

43. Turner, Jeffrey S., and Helms, Donald B. *Life Span Development*. Philadelphia: W. B. Saunders, 1979.

**44.** U.S. Department of Health and Human Services. *Promoting Health/ Preventing Disease: Objectives for the Nation.* Washington, DC: Government Printing Office, 1980.

**45.** Weinsier, Roland L., and Butterworth, C. E., Jr. *Handbook of Clinical Nutrition.* St. Louis: C. V. Mosby, 1981.

**46.** Whitney, Eleanor, and Hamilton, Eva May. *Understanding Nutrition.* St. Paul: West Publishing, 1977.

**47.** Williams, Sue Rodwell. *Nutrition and Diet Therapy.* 3rd ed. St. Louis: C. V. Mosby, 1977.

**48.** Wilson, Emery A., ed. *Nutrition in Pregnancy. Summary Report and Selected Papers from a Seminar for Clinical Nutritionists, May 19–21, 1980.* Lexington: University of Kentucky, 1980.

**49.** Wingate, M. B., *et al.* "Diseases Specific to Pregnancy." In *The Health Care of Women,* edited by S. L. Rommey *et al.* New York: McGraw-Hill, 1975.

**50.** Worthington-Roberts, Bonnie S.; Vermeersch, Joyce; and Williams, Sue R. *Nutrition in Pregnancy and Lactation.* 2nd ed. St. Louis: C. V. Mosby, 1981.

## Journals/Articles

**51.** American Academy of Pediatrics. "Breast-feeding." *Pediatrics* 62 (October 1978): 591–601.

**52.** Anderson, Garland D. "Nutrition in Pregnancy—1978." *Southern Medical Journal* 72 (October 1979): 1304–1314.

**53.** Barber, Hugh R. K. "Drugs During Pregnancy: Overview." *Symposia Reporter* 4 (May 1981): 1–2.

**54.** Barness, Lewis. "Infant Feeding: Benefits of Formulas." *The Professional Nutritionist* 12 (Summer 1980): 4–6.

**55.** Berg, Alan. "The Crisis in Infant Feeding Practices." *Nutrition Today* 12 (January/February 1977): 18–23.

**56.** Bowes, Watson A. "The Effect of Medications on the Lactating Mother and Her Infant." *Clinical Obstetrics and Gynecology* 23 (December 1980): 1073–79.

**57.** Brewer, T. "Role of Malnutrition in Pre-eclampsia and Eclampsia." *American Journal of Obstetrics and Gynecology* 125 (1976): 281–82.

**58.** Brody, Jane E. "Deficiencies of Vitamins." *New York Times Magazine,* March 29, 1981.

**59.** Brody, Jane E. "Feeding the Unborn: Some Diet Wisdom for Mothers-to-Be." *New York Times,* November 28, 1979.

**60.** Chung, R., *et al.* "Diet-Related Toxemia in Pregnancy." *American Journal of Clinical Nutrition* 32 (1979): 1902.

**61.** Churchill, John A., and Berendes, Heinz W. "Intelligence and Children Whose Mothers Had Acetonuria During Pregnancy." *Perinatal Factors Affecting Human Development* 185 (1969): 30–35.

**62.** Collins, Edith. "Non-Narcotic Analgesics During Pregnancy." *Symposia Reporter* 4 (May 1981): 8.

**63.** Cook, J. D., and Monsen, E. R. "Food Iron Absorption in Human Subjects." *American Journal of Clinical Nutrition* 29 (1976): 859.

**64.** Cunningham, A. S. "Morbidity in Breast-fed and Artificially Fed Infants, II." *Journal of Pediatrics* 95 (November 1979): 685.

**65.** *Diary Council Digest.* "Current Infant Feeding Practices." 51 (January–February 1980): 1–5.

**66.** *Dairy Council Digest.* "Food Faddism." 44 (January–February 1973): 1.

**67.** *Diabetes Forecast.* "Birthing Since Banting" 33 (September–October 1980): 29.

**68.** Disler, P. B., *et al.* "The Effect of Tea on Iron Absorption." *Gut* 16 (1975): 193.

**69.** Edidin, Deborah V., *et al.* "Resurgence of Nutritional Rickets Associated with Breastfeeding and Special Dietary Practices." *Pediatrics* 65 (February 1980): 232.

**70.** Edwards, Laura E., *et al.* "Pregnancy in the Underweight Woman: Course, Outcome, and Growth Patterns of the Infant." *American Journal of Obstetrics and Gynecology* 135 (1979): 297–302.

**71.** Enloe, Cortez F., Jr. "How Alcohol Affects the Developing Fetus." *Nutrition Today* 15 (September–October 1980): 12–16.

**72.** *Environmental Nutrition Newsletter.* "Questions from Our Readers." 4 (May 1981): 6.

**73.** Fairweather, D. V. I. "Nausea and Vomiting in Pregnancy." *American Journal of Obstetrics and Gynecology* 102 (September 1968): 135.

**74.** *FDA Consumer.* "Getting to the Seat of the Problem." 14 (September 1980): 18–23.

**75.** *FDA Consumer.* "A Primer on Dietary Minerals." September 1974. Reprinted as HEW Publication No. (FDA) 77-2070.

**76.** *FDA Drug Bulletin.* "Surgeon General's Advisory on Alcohol and Pregnancy." 11 (July 1981).

**77.** Fenner, Louise. "Salt Shakes Up Some of Us." *FDA Consumer* 14 (March 1980): 2–7.

**78.** Fielding, J. E. "Smoking and Pregnancy." *New England Journal of Medicine* 298 (February 1978): 337–39.

**79.** Fielding, J. E., and Yankauer, A. "The Pregnant Drinker." *American Journal of Public Health* 68 (1978): 836.

80. Filer, Lloyd J., Jr. "Maternal Nutrition in Lactation." *Clinics in Perinatology* 2 (September 1975): 353–60.

81. Finnegan, Loretta P. "Effects of Caffeine and Nicotine." *Symposia Reporter* 4 (May 1981): 20–21.

82. Fomon, S., and Strauss, R. G. "Nutritional Deficiency in Breastfed Infants." *New England Journal of Medicine* 299 (August 1978): 355.

83. Franz, Marion. "Nutritional Management in Diabetes and Pregnancy." *Diabetes Care* 1 (July–August 1978): 264–70.

84. Hare, J. W., and Solomon, E. K. "Giving Birth." *Diabetes Care* 34 (January–February 1981): 26–32.

85. Hecht, Annabel. "Advice on Breast-feeding and Drugs." *FDA Consumer* 13 (November 1979).

86. Hecht, Annabel. "Calcium: More Than Just the Strong Stuff of Bones." *FDA Consumer* 15 (July–August 1981): 14–17.

87. Herbert, Victor. "Pangamic Acid—Vitamin B-15, Fact or Fancy?" *The Professional Nutritionist* 11 (Winter 1979).

88. Higgins, Agnes C. "Nutritional Status and Outcome of Pregnancy." *Journal of the Canadian Dietetic Association* 37 (1976): 17–35.

89. Hill, Reba M.; Craig, Janice P.; *et al.* "Utilization of Over-the-Counter Drugs During Pregnancy." *Clinical Obstetrics and Gynecology* 20 (June 1977):381–93.

90. Hinds, Michael deCourcy. "Bottled Water a Health Aid? U.S. and Industry Agree: NO." *New York Times,* August 13, 1981.

91. Hopkins, Harold. "Next to Mother's Milk, There's Infant Formula." *FDA Consumer* 14 (July–August 1980):11–13.

92. Iber, Frank L. "Fetal Alcohol Syndrome." *Nutrition Today* 15 (September–October 1980): 4–11.

93. Jacobson, Howard N. "Diet and Pregnancy." *Nutrition and the M.D.* 6 (November 1980): 1–4.

94. Jacobson, Howard N. "Current Concepts in Nutrition: Diet in Pregnancy." *New England Journal of Medicine* 297 (November 1977):1051.

95. Jacobson, Howard N. "Nutrition and Pregnancy." *Journal of the American Dietetic Association* 60 (January 1972):26–29.

96. Jelliffe, Derrick B., *et al.* "The Mother-Child Dyad—Nutritional Aspects." *American Journal of Clinical Nutrition* 31 (August 1978): 1425–30.

97. Jelliffe, Derrick B., and Jelliffe, E. F. Patrice. " 'Breast Is Best': Modern Meanings." *New England Journal of Medicine* 297 (October 1977): 912–15.

98. Johnson, G. Timothy. "Anti-Nausea Drug OK for Pregnant Women." *Chicago Tribune,* May 20, 1981.

99. Jouganatos, D. M., and Gabbe, S. G. "Diabetes in Pregnancy: Changes and Current Management." *Journal of the American Dietetic Association* 73 (1978): 168.

100. Kaminetzky, Harold A., and Baker, Herman. "Micronutrients in Pregnancy." *Clinical Obstetrics and Gynecology* 20 (June 1977): 363–79.

100A. Kolata, Gina Bari. "Fetal Alcohol Advisory Debated." *Science* 214 (November 6, 1981): 642–645.

101. Lawson, John. "Current Views on the Management of Eclampsia." *Clinics in Obstetrics and Gynaecology* 4 (December 1977).

102. Lecos, Chris. "Caution Light on Caffeine." *FDA Consumer* 14 (October 1980): 6–9.

103. Liebman, Bonnie. "The Standard Fare Is Full of Fat: Salad Dressings." *Nutrition Action* 8 (October 1981): 12–13.

104. Marano, Hara. "Breast-feeding: New Evidence It's Far More than Nutrition." *Medical World News* 20 (February 1979).

105. Mata, L. "Breast-feeding: Main Promoter of Infant Health." *American Journal of Clinical Nutrition* 31 (1978):2058.

106. Mayer, Jean, and Dwyer, Johanna. "Pregnancy Do's and Don'ts." *Chicago Tribune*, March 1, 1979, p. 16.

107. Mayer, Jean, and Goldberg, Jeanne. "Will Vitamin $B_6$ Supplements Ease Morning Sickness and Nausea?" *Los Angeles Times*, January 29, 1981.

108. McMillan, Julia, Landaw, Stephen A.; and Oski, Frank A. "Iron Sufficiency in Breast-Fed Infants and the Availability of Iron from Human Milk." *Pediatrics* 58 (November 1976): 686–91.

109. Meyer, Mary B. "How Does Maternal Smoking Affect Birth Weight and Maternal Weight Gain?" *American Journal of Obstetrics and Gynecology* 131 (August 1978):888–93.

110. Meyer, Mary B., *et al.* "Perinatal Events Associated with Maternal Smoking During Pregnancy." *American Journal of Epidemiology* 103 (1976): 464.

111. Morrison, Margaret. "When the Baby's Life Is So Much Your Own . . ." *FDA Consumer* 13 (May 1979).

112. Mulcahy, R., and Knaggs, J. F. "Effect of Age, Parity, and Cigarette Smoking on Outcome of Pregnancy." *American Journal of Obstetrics and Gynecology* 101 (July 1968): 844–49.

113. Naeye, Richard L. "Effects of Maternal Cigarette Smoking on the Fetus and Placenta." *British Journal of Obstetrics and Gynecology* 80 (October 1978): 732–37.

114. Naeye, Richard L. "Weight Gain and the Outcome of Pregnancy." *American Journal of Obstetrics and Gynecology* 135 (September 1979): 3–9.

115. *New York Times*, "Reaching College Students in Print." January 16, 1978, p. 4.

116. *Nutrition and the M.D.* "The Pregnant Diabetic Patient." 6 (November 1980): 1–2.

117. *Nutrition Reviews.* "Maternal Weight Gain and the Outcome of Pregnancy." 37 (October 1979): 318–21.

118. *Nutrition Reviews.* "Morbidity in Breast-Fed and Artificially Fed Infants." 38 (March 1980):114–15.

119. Opp, Marcia. "Back to the Breast." *Family Style* 1 (March–April 1981):20.

120. *Pediatrics.* "Breast Feeding." Nutrition Committee of Canadian Paediatric Society and the Committee on Nutrition of the American Academy of Pediatrics (joint statement). 62 (1978): 591–601.

121. *Pediatrics.* "Committee on Nutrition: Commentary on Breast-Feeding and Infant Formulas, Including Proposed Standards for Formulas." 57 (1976): 278–85.

122. *Perinatal Developmental Medicine.* "The Diabetic Pregnancy and Its Outcome." 13 (June 1978):1–73.

123. Perkins, Richard P. "Management of the Hypertensive Pregnant Patient." *Clinics in Perinatology* 7 (September 1980).

124. Phillips, Margaret C., and Briggs, George M. "Symposium: Milk and Dairy Products for the American Diet." *Journal of Dairy Science* 58 (1975): 1751–63.

125. Pitkin, Roy M. "Calcium Metabolism in Pregnancy: A Review." *American Journal of Obstetrics and Gynecology* 121 (March 1975):724–35.

126. Pitkin, Roy M., *et al.* "Calcium Metabolism in Normal Pregnancy: A Longitudinal Study." *American Journal of Obstetrics and Gynecology* 133 (April 1979):781–90.

127. Pitkin, Roy M. "Maternal Nutrition: A Selective Review of Clinical Topics." *Obstetrics and Gynecology* 40 (December 1972):773–85.

128. Pitkin, Roy M. "Nutritional Support in Obstetrics and Gynecology." *Clinical Obstetrics and Gynecology* 19 (September 1976):489–513.

129. Pitkin, Roy M. "Vitamins and Minerals in Pregnancy." *Clinics in Perinatology* 2 (September 1975):221–32.

130. Pitkin, Roy M. "What's New in Maternal Nutrition?" *Nutrition News* 42 (April–May 1979):5–6.

131. Rudolph, Abraham M. "Effects of Nonsteroidal Anti-Inflammatory Drugs." *Symposia Reporter* 4 (May 1981):11–13.

132. Shank, R. E. "A Chink in Our Armor." *Nutrition Today* 5 (Summer 1970):2–11.

133. Sonstegard, Lois. "Pregnancy-Induced Hypertension: Prenatal Nursing Concerns." *American Journal of Maternal Child Nursing* 4 (March–April 1979):90–95.

134. Stearns, Genevieve. "Nutritional State of the Mother Prior to Conception." *Journal of the American Medical Association* 168 (November 1958):1655–59.

135. Stehbens, J. A., Baker, G. L., and Kitchell, M. "Outcome at Ages 1, 3, and 5 Years of Children Born to Diabetic Women." *American Journal of Obstetrics and Gynecology* 127 (February 1977):408.

136. Taylor, Flora. "Aspirin: America's Favorite Drug." *FDA Consumer* 14 (December 1980–January 1981):12–16.

137. Tichy, Anna M., and Chong, Dianne. "Placental Function and Its Role in Toxemia." *American Journal of Maternal Child Nursing* 4 (March–April 1979): 84–89.

138. Tompkins, Winslow T., Weihl, D. G., and Mitchell, R. "The Under-weight Patient as an Increased Obstetric Hazard." *American Journal of Obstetrics and Gynecology* 69 (January 1955):114–27.

139. Upton, Kim. "Caffeine Use Brews Health Controversy." *Chicago Sun-Times*, January 27, 1981, p. 37.

140. Varro, Barbara. "Substances That Can Slow Fetal Growth." *Chicago Sun-Times*, January 18, 1981.

141. Welt, S. I., and Crenshaw, M. C. "Concurrent Hypertension and Pregnancy." *Clinical Obstetrics and Gynecology* 21 (September 1978): 619.

142. White, Gregory J., and White, Mary Kerwin. "Breastfeeding and Drugs in Human Milk." *Veterinary and Human Toxicology* 22, Suppl. #1 (1980).

143. Whitehead, R. G. "Nutrition and Lactation." *Postgraduate Medical Journal* 55 (May 1979):303–10.

144. Winick, Myron. "Infant Nutrition: Formula or Breast Feeding?" *The Professional Nutritionist* 12 (Spring 1980):1–3.

145. Woodlin, G. B. "FDA Examines Caffeine." *Food Product Development* 15 (February 1981):48–50.

146. Worthington, Bonnie S. "Nutrition During Pregnancy, Lactation, and Oral Contraception." *Nursing Clinics of North America* 14 (June 1979):269–83.

147. Yaffe, Sumner J., and Filer, Lloyd J., Jr. "The Use and Abuse of Vitamin A." *Pediatrics* 48 (1971):655–56.


**Reports/Booklets**

148. American College of Obstetricians and Gynecologists, and American Dietetic Association. *Assessment of Maternal Nutrition*. Chicago: 1978.

149. American College of Obstetricians and Gynecologists. "Cesarean Birth." Patient Information Booklet. February 1981.

150. American Council on Science and Health. *The Health Effects of Caffeine: A Report by the American Council on Science and Health*. Summit, NJ: March 1981.

**150A.** American Council on Science and Health. *Alcohol Use During Pregnancy: A Report by the American/Council of Science and Health.* Summit, NJ: December 1981.

**151.** California State Department of Public Health. "Nutrition During Pregnancy and Lactation." Maternal and Child Health Branch. 1975.

**151A.** Committee on Nutrition of the Mother and Preschool Child. Food and Nutrition Board, National Research Council. *Nutrition Services in Prenatal Care.* National Academy Press. Washington, DC: 1981.

**151B.** Institute of Nutrition. *Caffeine.* Institute of Nutrition, University of North Carolina: May 1981.

**152.** March of Dimes Birth Defects Foundation. "Be Good to Your Baby Before It Is Born." White Plains, NY: 1980.

**153.** March of Dimes Birth Defects Foundation. "D*A*T*A*: Drugs, Alcohol, Tobacco Abuse During Pregnancy." White Plains, NY: 1980.

**154.** March of Dimes Birth Defects Foundation. "Pregnant? Before You Drink, Think . . ." White Plains, NY: 1979.

**155.** Ministry of Health. "Baby's Best Chance." Nutrition Division, Province of British Columbia. Victoria, British Columbia: 1978.

**156.** Ministry of Health. "Nutrition: Eating for a Baby." Nutrition Division, Province of British Columbia. Victoria, British Columbia: 1978.

**157.** Ministry of Health. "Nutrition: Infant Nutrition Guide." Nutrition Division, Province of British Columbia. Victoria, British Columbia: 1978.

**158.** National Academy of Sciences. *Maternal Nutrition and the Course of Pregnancy: Report of the Committee on Maternal Nutrition.* National Research Council. Washington, DC: 1970.

**159.** The Nutrition Foundation, Inc. *The Feeding of the Very Young: An Approach to Determination of Policies. A Report of the International Advisory Group on Infant and Child Feeding.* New York: 1978.

**160.** State of Illinois, Governor's Citizens Advisory Council on Alcoholism. "Fetal Alcohol Syndrome Work Group: For Your Baby's Sake, Don't Drink!" Chicago: 1980.

**161.** Tsang, Reginald C. "On Developmental Nutrition: Calcium and Phosphorus, Number 11." University of Cincinnati. Cincinnati: 1975.

**162.** U.S. Department of Agriculture and U.S. Department of Health, Education and Welfare. "Nutrition and Your Health: Dietary Guidelines for Americans." Home and Garden Bulletin No. 232. Washington, D.C.: 1980.

**163.** U.S. Department of Health, Education and Welfare, Public Health Services. *Symposium on Human Lactation.* Washington, DC: Government Printing Office, 1976.

**164.** U.S. Department of Health, Education and Welfare. "The Health Consequences of Smoking." Public Health Service. Government Printing Office. Washington, DC: 1975.

**165.** U.S. Department of Health and Human Services. "Should I Drink?" National Institute on Alcohol Abuse and Alcoholism. DHHS Publication No. (ADM) 80-919. Rockville, MD: 1980.

**166.** Watson, Kay. "Nutrition for You and Your Baby." Royal Victoria Hospital. Montreal, Quebec: 1977.

**167.** Woodruff, Calvin. "Supplementary Foods for Infants." *Contemporary Nutrition*. General Mills, Inc. Minneapolis: MN 1980.

**168.** World Health Organization. *Smoking and Its Effects on Health: A Report of a WHO Expert Committee.* World Health Organization Technical Report Series No. 568. Geneva, Switzerland: 1975.

## Speeches/Tapes/Communications

**169.** Edidin, Dr. Deborah V. Assistant Professor of Pediatrics, Pritzker School of Medicine, University of Chicago. Interview, May 12, 1981. Chicago, Illinois.

**170.** Filer, Dr. Lloyd J., Jr. Tanner Lecture to the Chicago Section of the Institute of Food Technologists, May 11, 1981. Chicago, Illinois.

**171.** Frederiksen, Dr. Marilyn. Maternal-Fetal Specialist, Prentice Women's Hospital. October 19, 1981. Chicago, Illinois.

**172.** Higgins, Agnes. Lecture to the Society for Nutrition Education. July 8, 1980. Montreal, Quebec.

**172A.** Jacobson, Howard N. Director, Institute of Nutrition, University of North Carolina. Personal telephone communication. November 10, 1981.

**173.** Neifert, Dr. Mary Ann. Lecture at International Conference of the La Leche League, July 24, 1981. Chicago, Illinois.

**174.** Newton, Niles. Lecture within workshop sponsored by the Rockford Regional Perinatal Center, December 18, 1980. Rockford, Illinois.

**175.** Mullen, Dr. Joseph. Lecture at symposium sponsored by the Chicago Nutrition Association, April 30, 1980. Chicago, Illinois.

**176.** Observation by co-author Mary Abbott Hess.

# Index

247

## About the Authors

Mary Abbott Hess and Anne Elise Hunt are partners in Hess and Hunt, Inc., a firm specializing in the development of nutrition communication materials. Mary Abbott Hess, a registered dietitian, is a nationally known authority on nutrition. She is a former Associate Professor at Mundelein College in Chicago and has served on the faculty of several Chicago-area nursing schools as nutrition co-ordinator. She and her husband, Peter, an attorney, have two daughters: Rachel, age twelve, and Leslie, age ten.

Anne Elise Hunt is a home economist and food journalist. She is a former food editor of *Sphere* (now *Cuisine*) magazine, and was an account executive for a Chicago public relations firm specializing in food product communications. Anne's husband, Bruce, teaches continuing professional education at the University of Chicago. They have three daughters: Lisa, age twenty; Jennifer, age eighteen; and Mary, age fifteen.